LIVING
HEART
IN THE 21ST CENTURY

MICHAEL E. DeBAKEY, MD
ANTONIO M. GOTTO JR., MD, DPhil

THE

LIVING
HEART

IN THE 21st CENTURY

FOREWORD BY
GEORGE P. NOON, MD

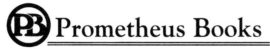 Prometheus Books

59 John Glenn Drive
Amherst, New York 14228–2119

Published 2012 by Prometheus Books

Cover image © 2012 Media Bakery
Cover design by Grace M. Conti-Zilsberger

Inquiries should be addressed to
Prometheus Books
59 John Glenn Drive
Amherst, New York 14228–2119
VOICE: 716–691–0133
FAX: 716–691–0137
WWW.PROMETHEUSBOOKS.COM

16 15 14 13 12   5 4 3 2 1

Library of Congress Cataloging-in-Publication Data

DeBakey, Michael E. (Michael Ellis), 1908–2008.
    The living heart in the 21st century / by Michael E. DeBakey and Antonio M. Gotto Jr.
        p. cm.
    Includes bibliographical references and index.
    ISBN 978–1–61614–563–7 (pbk. : alk. paper)
    ISBN 978–1–61614–564–4 (ebook)
    1. Heart—Diseases—Treatment—Popular works. 2. Cardiovascular system—
Diseases—Treatment—Popular works. I. Gotto, Antonio M. II. Title.

RC672.D412 2012
616.12—dc23

                                                                2011050593

Printed in the United States of America on acid-free paper

The authors dedicate this book to our wives,
Katrin DeBakey and Anita Gotto,
and daughters,
Olga DeBakey, Jennifer Gotto Roberts, Gillian Gotto, and Teresa Teague,
who encouraged and supported us throughout our careers.

CONTENTS

FOREWORD

Drs. Michael DeBakey and Antonio Gotto have long been instrumental in developing research programs, prevention strategies, and innovative treatment of heart and vascular disease. In 1977, they published the first edition of the Living Heart series to provide the lay reader with information to better understand signs and symptoms, diagnoses, and treatments of the specific conditions comprising cardiovascular disease. Since then, remarkable progress has been made in research, prevention, diagnosis, and treatment of cardiovascular disease.

Dr. DeBakey and associates have made outstanding contributions in devising and refining operative procedures for heart and vascular disease. In 1932, as a medical student, Dr. DeBakey developed a roller pump that later became an integral component of the first heart-lung machine, which Dr. John Gibbons devised and first used clinically in 1950. In 1953, Dr. DeBakey performed a resection (surgical removal) of an abdominal aortic aneurysm (a blood-filled sac caused by the stretching of the walls of the aorta) and replacement with a cadaver aortic homograft. The following year, he performed the first successful carotid endarterectomy (surgical removal of atherosclerotic plaque within the carotid arteries in the neck). In 1954, he developed the Dacron™ graft, which became the standard arterial prosthesis for blood vessel replacement and bypass procedures. Aneurysms located at four different sections of the aorta, the large artery originating from the heart, were successfully removed and replaced with DeBakey Dacron grafts (ascending aorta, arch, descending thoracic aorta, and thoracoabdominal aorta).

In 1964, Dr. DeBakey and associates performed the first successful autogenous saphenous vein coronary artery bypass (heart bypass surgery using a vein from the patient's own leg to reroute blood flow). That was followed two years later by the first successful human implantation of an LVAD (left ventricular assist device) for heart failure after cardiac surgery. In 1968, Dr. DeBakey and associates performed the first donor multiorgan harvest and transplanted the donor's heart, lung, and two kidneys in four different patients. In 1998, the first implantation of the MicroMed DeBakey Noon VAD demonstrated for the first time that a patient could live a normal life without pulsatile flow (blood is propelled continuously throughout the circulation without producing a measurable pulse).

I first met Dr. Michael E. DeBakey in 1958 when I was a medical student at Baylor University College of Medicine (BUCM), where I worked part-time on research projects in the department of surgery, including aortic dissecting aneurysms. After graduating from medical school, I completed my general surgery and thoracic surgery residencies under Dr. DeBakey at BUCM, and in 1967 I joined Dr. DeBakey's department of surgery and worked with him thereafter. I witnessed or participated in many of his firsts and other achievements. We traveled to the USSR in 1973 to operate on academician Mstislav Keldysh, the leading Soviet scientist, and to Russia in 1998 to participate in the care of President Boris Yeltsin in Moscow. We cared for the rich and poor from around the world, including presidents, royalty, celebrities, and ordinary citizens.

Dr. DeBakey was very active into his nineties. He had major responsibilities in Houston, and he traveled and lectured around the world. His health and stamina were remarkable. On December 31, 2005, he was working in his library at home when he experienced a sudden onset of severe right-sided neck pain. He thought he was having a myocardial infarction (heart attack) or a dissecting aneurysm (tearing within the walls of an artery). He remained at home for his initial evaluation, which showed no evidence of myocardial infarction. On January 3, 2006, a CT scan demonstrated a 5.7 cm DeBakey Type II dissecting aneurysm. (In 1954, Dr. DeBakey had first performed a resection and a graft replacement of a dissecting aneurysm. He later classified them as DeBakey Type I, II, and III.) He elected no surgery at the time the diagnosis was established, preferring to continue with his medical regimen and close follow-ups. On January 6, 2006, Dr. DeBakey lectured to the Academy of Medicine, Engineering, and Science of Texas on "Mechanical Circulatory Assistance." The audience had no idea of his serious condition.

Dr. DeBakey's care was continued at home until January 23, 2006, when he was hospitalized for closer observation. The aneurysm had increased in size to 6.78 cm. The intramural hematoma (accumulation of blood within the artery wall) had further increased on January 24. Dr. DeBakey elected to continue observation. A category II life-sustaining treatment directive was signed by one of his physicians on January 29, 2006, but never by Dr. DeBakey. When I questioned him about what he would want us to do if he were not able to make a decision regarding his care, he responded, "Do whatever is necessary." On February 9, 2006, a magnetic resonance angiogram (MRA) showed further increase in the size of the aneurysm to 7.798 cm, with an increase in pericardial effusion and pleural effusion (accumulation of fluid around the heart and lungs), greater on the left than the right. These changes were significant and suggested bleeding from the aneurysm with high risk for rupture. Evidence of a cerebral lesion on the MRA proved to be an artifact (erroneous image) on a follow-up CT scan. Dr. DeBakey had been sedated for the MRA.

The patient's status and therapeutic options were discussed with the family. The family, which included his wife, daughter, three sons, and two sisters, decided on surgery, aware of the risks and alternatives. His wife signed an operative permit. The anesthesiologist was reluctant to participate in the surgical procedure, and the family requested another anesthesiologist. The hospital ethics committee was summoned to make a final decision and resolve the issue regarding his care, and it was agreed that we could proceed with surgery. We surgically removed a Type II dissecting aneurysm of the ascending aorta and replaced it with a DeBakey Dacron graft. The aortic valve was reattached. The operation was performed with the use of cardiopulmonary bypass (stopping the heart and maintaining blood circulation with a heart-lung machine), profound hypothermia, and circulatory arrest. He was weaned from cardiopulmonary bypass and transferred to the intensive care unit. Postoperatively, when questioned on multiple occasions, Dr. DeBakey stated he agreed with the decision for surgery and was glad to be alive. During his postoperative course, he required temporary support with an intra-aortic balloon pump, dialysis, tracheostomy, and gastrostomy, which were used from days to months. Throughout this period, his mental status was never impaired.

With the superb care of his medical team, nurses, physical therapist, and family, he was finally able to be discharged from the hospital on September 2, 2006. Following his discharge, he resumed his work schedule. He would go to his office during workdays after early morning physical therapy. He walked every day but mainly used an electric wheelchair. At least once a week, he met with his medical team to review his progress and care. An avid gardener, he would bring his heirloom tomatoes and peppers and distribute them to the team. He continued a busy schedule, consulting and attending meetings at the Texas Medical Center in Houston, where he participated in the groundbreaking of the Michael E. DeBakey Museum and Library.

On April 21, 2008, he traveled to Washington, DC, to receive the Congressional Gold Medal from President George W. Bush. Dr. DeBakey felt honored to receive this high award and the medallion designed for him. The inscription on the medallion over an image of a heart and blood vessels reads, "The pursuit of excellence has been my objective in life."

Dr. DeBakey continued his office work and activities, looking forward to celebrating his one hundredth birthday. On July 11, 2008, he was visited at home by Dr. Gotto, who discussed with him the new edition of *The Living Heart*. Later in the day I also visited with Dr. DeBakey, and we had a snack together. I had gumbo with peppers from his garden, and he had ice cream. When I was leaving, I told him I was going to my grandson's baseball game and would be vacationing for a week in Aspen. He said, "Best of luck to your grandson, and I will see you when you return from Aspen." Within two hours, he unexpectedly collapsed and could not be resuscitated. He would have been one-hundred years old in fifty-eight days, on September 7, 2008. God bless you, Dr. DeBakey; we miss you dearly.

George P. Noon, MD
Professor of Surgery
Chief, Division of Transplant and Assist Devices
Michael E. DeBakey Department of Surgery
Baylor College of Medicine
Houston, Texas

PREFACE

The fight against heart disease begins with information. In the movies and on television, heart attacks are dramatic—a person who seems completely healthy suddenly keels over on the floor. In reality, heart disease is an insidious process that can develop over a lifetime. However, there are concrete steps that you can take to prevent heart disease or to treat it if it does develop.

The first book I wrote with Dr. Michael DeBakey, *The Living Heart*, was published in 1977. Since then, we have collaborated on a series of related books for patients and general readers. These books have explained how heart disease develops, how to eat healthily, and how best to treat various heart conditions.

Cardiovascular medicine has seen major advances since the original *Living Heart* book was published. In the United States, mortality rates from coronary heart disease have decreased by more than 40 percent in both men and women since 1980.[1] However, cardiovascular disease continues to be the leading cause of death in the United States, with one death from heart disease occurring every thirty-nine seconds. Still, death rates from cardiovascular disease have decreased by 28 percent from 1997 to 2007.[2] About one-half of the decrease in mortality over the past several decades is due to recent improvements in cardiac surgery and medication.[3] The other half is due to improved control of risk factors for cardiovascular disease, such as high cholesterol, high blood pressure, cigarette smoking, and physical inactivity.

Although heart disease remains a major health threat, we have learned a lot over the past three decades about what causes it, how to detect it earlier, and how to treat it more effectively. *The Living Heart in the Twenty-First Century* has been completely revised and updated to present the latest information on cardiovascular prevention, diagnosis, and treatment. It contains essential knowledge and lifesaving tips distilled from our combined years of experience treating cardiology patients. We hope that this book will be a resource for patients and general readers who want to improve or maintain their cardio-vascular health, as well as for relatives, friends, and caretakers of people with heart disease. Don't feel the need to read the book straight through. It has been designed so that you can easily find as much information on a particular topic as you need. Some important and relevant information may be repeated throughout various sections. Read the sections that you feel most apply to you.

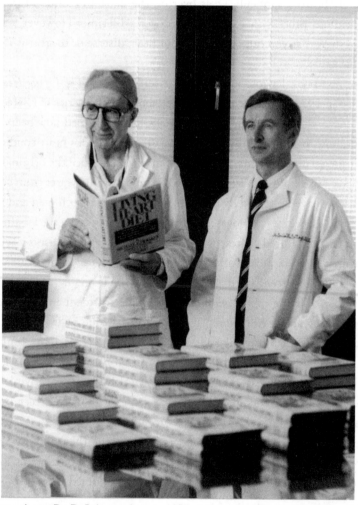

This photo shows Dr. DeBakey and me in 1984 at the release for our book *The Living Heart Diet. Photograph courtesy of the author.*

The most common form of heart disease is coronary heart disease, which is caused by atherosclerosis and can often lead to the chest pains of angina or to a heart attack. The first chapter contains information about how atherosclerosis develops and about the relationship between cholesterol and atherosclerosis. Prevention of coronary heart disease focuses on controlling risk factors, including diet, exercise, smoking, high cholesterol, high blood pressure, and obesity. Chapter 2 covers the latest guidelines on reducing cardiovascular risk, explains their scientific rationale, and provides advice on how to translate this information to your own life. Chapter 3 explains how doctors detect, diagnose, and treat coronary heart disease if it does occur so that patients can take charge of their own health care and communicate more effectively with their medical providers. It covers recent advances in medical imaging that allow physicians to more accurately visualize the heart and blood vessels and to perform delicate diagnostic tests and interventions. Chapter 4 covers the major forms of atherosclerotic disease, including angina, heart attack, peripheral artery disease, and stroke, while chapter 5 describes the latest innovations in treatment for these conditions.

Most popular books on heart disease focus on prevention and treatment of heart attacks, but arrhythmias, heart failure, and valvular disease also commonly affect the heart. *The Living Heart in the Twenty-First Century* describes how these other conditions are recognized and most effectively addressed today. Dietary and lifestyle recommendations, medication and surgery, and the newest implantable devices for arrhythmias, heart failure, and valvular disease are presented in chapters 6, 7, and 8, respectively. Finally, chapter 9 offers a glimpse of the exciting advances in cardiovascular medicine that the future holds.

We hope that you find this book helpful as you learn how to reduce your cardiovascular risk; why cardiologists offer the advice they do; and which medications, tests, and procedures are the most effective. In the twenty-first century, the fight against heart disease begins with information.

Antonio M. Gotto Jr., MD, DPhil
Stephen and Suzanne Weiss Dean and Professor of Medicine
December 2011
Weill Cornell Medical College
New York, New York

CHAPTER 1
CHOLESTEROL AND ATHEROSCLEROSIS
The New Biology

Oone of the most frequent causes of heart disease is *atherosclerosis*.
Atherosclerosis is a lifelong process that leads to the thickening and
hardening of artery walls. It is the underlying cause of nearly three-fourths of
all cardiovascular deaths. *Atherosclerotic plaques*, also called *lesions*, can develop
in the coronary arteries that surround the heart muscle and provide it with
blood (see figure 1.1). These plaques reduce the flow of blood and oxygen to
the heart, which can cause the chest pain or discomfort of *angina*. In more
severe cases of coronary heart disease, the plaques entirely block the flow of
blood to the heart, or they rupture, producing large blood clots that can then
cut off the heart's blood supply. In both instances, the result is a heart attack,
or what doctors call a *myocardial infarction*.

Heart attacks are a very common form of heart disease. According to the
American Heart Association, one heart attack occurs approximately every
twenty-five seconds in the United States.[1] Every minute, a person dies from
one. In one year, approximately 785,000 Americans will have a first attack,
while about 470,000 will have a repeat attack. Many of these events can be
prevented by implementing healthy lifestyle changes and by controlling risk
factors for atherosclerotic vascular disease.

A heart attack is just one of the events that can occur due to atherosclerosis. Atherosclerosis can also develop in any of the major arteries and in
the aorta, the large vessel that carries blood away from the heart (see figures
1.2a, 1.2b, and 1.2c). Plaques gradually constrict these arteries, and they can
rupture, leading to subsequent clot formation. Clots that become lodged in

the carotid arteries in the neck or the cerebral arteries in the brain can block blood flow to the brain, causing a *stroke* or *transient ischemic attack* (TIA). In addition, plaques can reduce the flow of blood and oxygen to surrounding tissues, which may eventually die. Atherosclerosis that develops in the femoral arteries of the leg or in the brachial arteries of the arms, called *peripheral artery disease* (PAD), can cause pain, decreased function, and in severe cases, gangrene leading to amputation. Atherosclerosis of the renal arteries in the kidney can cause high blood pressure and eventual kidney failure. Finally, the consequences of atherosclerosis can lead to arrhythmias (disorders of heart rate or rhythm), heart failure, and other conditions affecting the heart.

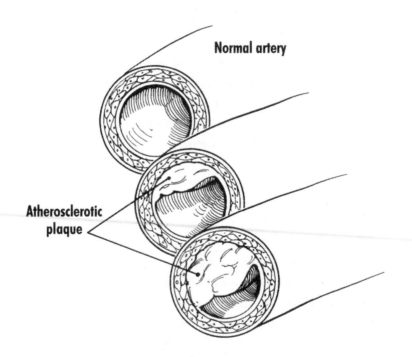

Figure 1.1. An atherosclerotic plaque develops in an artery and can reduce blood flow to organs and tissues. *Illustration created by Herbert R. Smith Jr.*

Understanding how *coronary heart disease* (CHD) and atherosclerosis develop is the first step in prevention. Many people in the twenty-first-century United States have high-fat, sedentary lifestyles that greatly increase the risk of developing atherosclerosis. However, atherosclerosis is not just a modern disease. Evidence of atherosclerosis has been found in Egyptian mummies dating from the third millennium BCE and in Peruvian remains from the first millennium BCE. The difference is that now, in the twenty-first century, we understand how and why atherosclerosis develops, as well as key strategies for prevention. This chapter highlights the major concepts about atherosclerosis that have emerged after more than a century of scientific research and due to recent advances in molecular biology. The story begins with cholesterol.

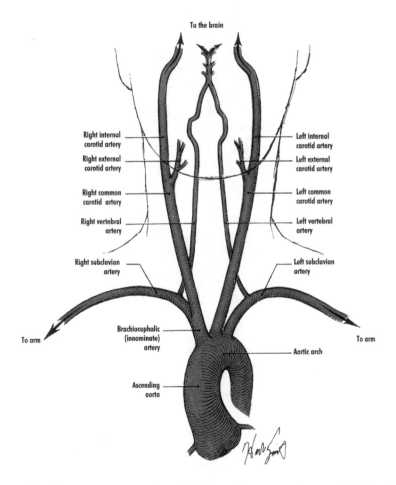

Figure 1.2a. Three major arteries branch off from the aortic arch to supply the head and arms with blood. *Illustration created by Herbert R. Smith Jr.*

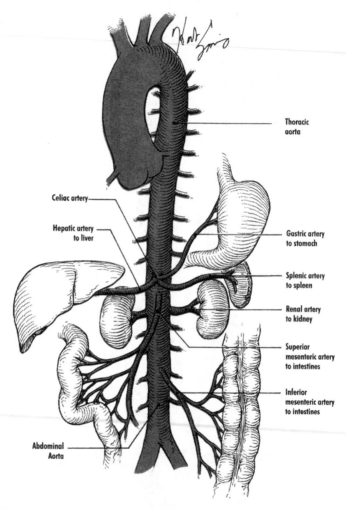

Thoracic
aorta

Celiac artery

Hepatic artery
to liver

Gastric artery
to stomach

Splenic artery
to spleen

Renal artery
to kidney

Superior
mesenteric artery
to intestines

Inferior
mesenteric artery
to intestines

Abdominal
Aorta

Figure 1.2b. Branches arise from the aorta in the chest and abdomen to supply blood to the major organs. *Illustration created by Herbert R. Smith Jr.*

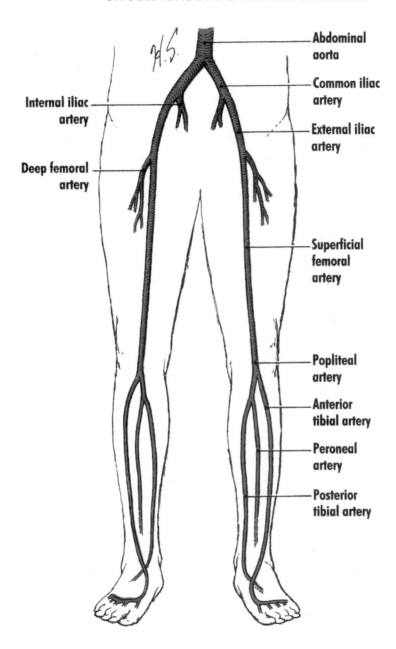

Figure 1.2c. The abdominal aorta branches into the iliac arteries to supply blood to the pelvis, thighs, and legs. *Illustration created by Herbert R. Smith Jr.*

WHY CHOLESTEROL?

In 1904, a German pathologist named Felix Marchand first proposed the term "atherosclerosis" to describe a process that nineteenth-century physicians were aware of but did not yet understand.[2] Marchand chose this name because of the appearance of the arteries he examined: "athero" is the Greek root for "gruel" or "porridge," while "sclerosis" is the root for "hardening." His choice emphasized the resemblance between the fatty atherosclerotic plaques found within hardened arteries and porridge. At the time, physicians did not know what material these soft, pulpy deposits consisted of, or what effect they might have on the body.

In 1913, scientists got their first real clue when a Russian scientist named Nikolai Anichkov fed rabbits cholesterol purified from egg yolks and was able to produce the same gruel-like deposits found in human arteries.[3] Anichkov also determined that the amount of cholesterol fed to the rabbits was related to the size and number of plaques that developed. Scientists did not fully recognize the significance of his findings until decades later. Now, however, it is clear that cholesterol is a major component of atherosclerotic lesions and that high levels of cholesterol in the blood, or *plasma*, can cause atherosclerosis and its many complications.

In the middle of the twentieth century, researchers studying large populations discovered a relationship between saturated fat consumption, total cholesterol levels, and heart disease. In the 1950s, the Seven Countries Study found that high consumption of saturated fat in countries such as the United States and Finland led to increased blood cholesterol levels and to much higher rates of heart disease, as compared to countries with low saturated fat consumption, such as Japan, Greece, and Italy.[4] In the 1960s, the Ni-Hon-San study examined men of Japanese descent who were living in Japan, Honolulu, and San Francisco.[5] It showed that cholesterol levels and heart disease all increased as diets became more Westernized and consumption of saturated fat increased. Japanese men living in San Francisco were found to have more heart attacks than those living in Honolulu and more than those living in Japan. Both the Seven Countries Study and the Ni-Hon-San study show that different populations can vary greatly in terms of their cholesterol levels and that these differences are mostly due to diet and lifestyle, not genetics. Other population studies, including the Framingham Heart Study, which began in 1948 in Massachusetts, have further verified the relationship between elevated blood cholesterol and coronary heart disease.[6] In general, these trials have established that each 1 percent increase in total blood cholesterol leads to an approximate 2 percent increase in risk for coronary heart disease events.[7]

WHAT IS CHOLESTEROL?

Cholesterol belongs to a group of naturally occurring molecules called *lipids*. The term "lipid" is often used to refer to fats, but lipids are actually a class of molecules, including fats, oils, waxes, and sterols, that can be dissolved in other fats, oils, and lipids but not in water (they are "lipophilic"). A major function of lipids is energy storage, which is how we commonly think of fats and oils. Other functions of lipids include maintaining the structure of cell membranes and regulating a wide variety of cellular activities, especially those that involve molecular signaling.

Cholesterol is a simple lipid. (Because of its chemical structure, it is also classified as an alcohol and as a form of *steroid* called a sterol.) *Fatty acids*, which are derived from animal and vegetable fats and oils, are another type of simple lipid. Omega fatty acids, for example, are most commonly found in fish. *Trans* fatty acids are a kind of processed plant oil sometimes used in commercial food preparation. Complex lipids include triglycerides, cholesteryl esters, and phospholipids. *Triglycerides* store energy in the body and are the primary components of vegetable oils and animal fats. Most fat in the human body and in food is in the form of triglycerides. *Cholesteryl ester* is a molecule of cholesterol that has undergone a chemical process called esterification that makes it easier to transport in the blood. Most of the cholesterol in the bloodstream exists in the form of cholesteryl esters. *Phospholipids* are an important component of cell membranes and of *lipoproteins*, which are specialized macromolecules (very large molecules) that transport cholesterol in the blood.

Too much cholesterol in the blood can lead to atherosclerosis, plaque formation, and heart disease, but cholesterol is essential to all animal life and is naturally synthesized by all animals. It plays a number of roles in the human body (see table 1.1). Most importantly, cholesterol is a major component of cell membranes and helps to maintain membrane fluidity. It is needed to form bile acids, which aid in the digestion and absorption of fat in the intestines. In addition, it is the main precursor for vitamin D and for the steroid hormones, including progesterone, estrogen, and testosterone. Cholesterol also plays roles in the conduction of nerve impulses and in cell signaling processes. Without cholesterol, the body would not be able to function on many different levels. Not surprisingly, a highly complex system has evolved to regulate the amount of cholesterol that is present at any given time in the bloodstream and available for transport to different parts of the body.

Table 1.1. Functions of Cholesterol in the Body

- Important component of cell membranes
  - Maintains membrane structure and fluidity
  - Helps transport substances into the cell
  - Facilitates communication between cells, including nerve cells
- Forms bile acid to digest food
- Precursor to vitamin D and steroid hormones

Cholesterol is carried in the blood mostly in the form of cholesteryl ester by lipoproteins, which are composed of both lipids and proteins. Lipoproteins contain some free cholesterol, but their major lipid components are cholesteryl esters, triglycerides, and phospholipids in varying concentrations. Lipoproteins are classified according to density in five major categories: high-density lipoprotein (HDL), intermediate-density lipoprotein (IDL), low-density lipoprotein (LDL), very low-density lipoprotein (VLDL), and chylomicrons (see figure 1.3). When doctors measure your cholesterol levels, they are determining the relative quantities of various lipoproteins and their components present in the blood at that moment. You may already be aware of HDL cholesterol (HDL-C), the "good" cholesterol, and LDL cholesterol (LDL-C), the "bad" cholesterol. (The "C" refers to the amount of cholesterol carried by HDL and LDL lipoproteins.) In order to understand what makes these types of cholesterol "good" or "bad," we need to go into a little more biological detail.

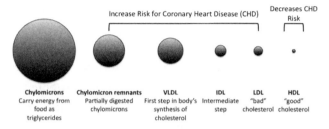

Figure 1.3. The five major categories of lipoproteins, plus chylomicron remnants, transport cholesterol and other lipids throughout the body in the blood. They each have a different relationship to atherosclerosis. (Drawing not to scale.) *Figure courtesy of the author.*

BASICS OF LIPID METABOLISM

The body synthesizes its own cholesterol, and in addition, cholesterol is acquired through the diet. When you consume a meal, the small intestines absorb only some of the cholesterol contained in the food, and the rest is excreted as waste. There is a wide variation among individuals in how much cholesterol tends to be absorbed by the intestines. These variations are probably determined in large part by genetics. Depending on how much cholesterol is absorbed from dietary sources, the body increases or decreases the amount of cholesterol it synthesizes so that cholesterol levels in the blood remain relatively constant.

Following a meal, the cholesterol that is absorbed into intestinal cells is packaged, along with triglycerides, as chylomicrons, which are extremely large lipoproteins not associated with atherosclerosis or heart disease. (Patients are asked to fast before having their cholesterol tested because the triglycerides present in chylomicrons following a meal can affect the accuracy of the measurements.) Chylomicrons are then transported through the lymphatic circulation (a subset of the circulatory system that helps maintain fluid balance) from the intestines and introduced into the bloodstream via the thoracic duct (a part of the lymphatic system located in the chest). The blood then circulates chylomicrons to tissues in various parts of the body where they are broken down to smaller particles known as chylomicron remnants. As they are broken down, chylomicrons release free fatty acids, which are either used by muscles immediately for energy or are converted to triglycerides to be stored as fat. The chylomicron remnants return to the liver with their remaining loads of cholesterol, most of which is then excreted by the intestines as waste. Unlike chylomicrons themselves, chylomicron remnants can contribute to the formation of atherosclerotic plaques, and a delay in digesting and removing them from the body is associated with an increased risk of coronary heart disease.

Along with the intestines, the liver is a key organ that maintains a balance of cholesterol within the blood. In addition to clearing the dietary cholesterol that is delivered by chylomicron remnants, the liver synthesizes the cholesterol needed to maintain the body's normal functioning. It can also take the cholesterol it produces out of the circulation. The entire process is one of continual synthesis, removal, and excretion.

The first step in the body's synthesis of cholesterol is the production of very low-density lipoprotein (VLDL) by the liver. VLDL has a high content of triglycerides, and it circulates in the blood in order to transport energy to various tissues throughout the body. VLDL can also be converted to intermediate-density lipoprotein (IDL), which is then converted to LDL. As VLDL is converted to IDL and then to LDL, it becomes increasingly enriched in cholesterol (in the form of cholesteryl esters) and depleted of triglycerides, resulting in progressively smaller and denser lipoprotein particles. LDL is the primary carrier of cholesterol in the blood, and LDL-C has deservedly gained a reputation as the "bad" cholesterol. VLDL, IDL, and LDL all promote atherosclerosis because they contain a protein called *apolipoprotein B* (apo B). Chylomicrons contain a different form of apo B, about one-half the size of that found in the other lipoproteins. LDL is the most important and the most commonly measured of the lipoproteins containing apo B. Scientists believe that primarily LDL and modified forms of LDL penetrate the walls of arteries, which is a key step in the formation of atherosclerotic plaques. If levels of LDL-C in the blood become too high, atherosclerosis starts to develop.

HOW DOES ATHEROSCLEROSIS DEVELOP?

When arteries are healthy, they have strong, flexible walls and a smooth inner lining. Atherosclerosis is a disease of the *intima*, or the innermost layer, of the arterial wall. Arteries have three layers: a thick, flexible outer wall called the *adventitia*; a middle, elastic layer called the *media*, which contains smooth muscle cells and is capable of constriction and relaxation; and the intima (see figure 1.4). The intima consists of a thin layer of endothelial cells, called the *endothelium*, that are directly exposed to blood flow through the *lumen*, or the inner space of the artery. A thin, internal elastic membrane separates the intima and the media. The *vasa vasorum* are a network of small blood vessels that supply large vessels.

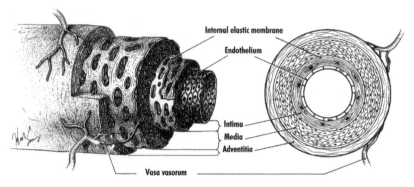

Figure 1.4. An artery has three layers of different types of cells. *Illustration created by Herbert R. Smith Jr.*

In the past, it was believed that atherosclerotic plaques developed progressively, with excess cholesterol in the blood gradually accumulating and leading to bigger and bigger plaques. Contemporary research now indicates that atherosclerosis may be considered a type of inflammatory disease involving many different steps.[8] The disease develops depending on the balance between LDL cholesterol, which is deposited *into* atherosclerotic plaques, and HDL, the "good" cholesterol responsible for transporting lipid back *out of* the plaque.

Scientists have long debated what the initiating step in the atherosclerotic process might be. What occurs in the arterial wall that causes cholesterol to accumulate and plaques to form in the first place? Generally, lipoproteins such as LDL flow in and out of the arterial wall, but in atherosclerosis, something occurs that makes their behavior different from normal. For the past few decades, scientists have believed that atherosclerosis begins as a "response to injury."[9] According to this theory, LDL particles penetrate the endothelium, causing damage to the surface of the arterial wall. This initial injury triggers a dysfunctional and inflammatory response within the vessel wall, which then starts the atherosclerotic process. The effects of cigarette smoking, high blood pressure, and diabetes can also damage the endothelium and accelerate the atherosclerotic process.

This view has since been modified to further explain why some lipoproteins cause damage to the arterial wall, while others do not. In 1995, researchers proposed a "response to retention" theory.[10] They hypothesized that the first step in the atherosclerotic process occurs when LDL particles penetrate the endothelium and then become *trapped* in the arterial wall. Apo B particles in LDL are believed to bind to molecules called *proteoglycans*, which normally provide structural support within the arterial wall.[11] LDL is then "retained" within the intima, where it can subsequently injure the endothelium and cause dysfunction. Although VLDL and IDL also contain apo B, LDL particles are smaller and may be more likely to penetrate the endothelium and bind to proteoglycans than larger lipoproteins.

The retention of LDL particles within the arterial wall leads to *inflammation* and *oxidation*, states that are believed to be especially conducive to atherosclerosis (see figure 1.5). A cascade of inflammatory molecules is produced, which makes the area "sticky" and attracts more LDL to the intima to be retained. Immune cells called *monocytes* and *T cells* are also attracted and drawn through the endothelium into the arterial wall. As LDL begins to accumulate, it can become chemically modified. The most common form of modification is called *oxidation*, which occurs through contact with unstable molecules called free radicals. Oxidized LDL is much more damaging to the arterial wall than regular LDL, and its presence triggers a heightened inflammatory and immune response that further attracts LDL and monocytes.

Recently it was theorized that antioxidants, which are abundant in fruits and vegetables, might be able to inhibit atherosclerosis and have beneficial effects on other diseases, including cancer. However, research to date has not shown that antioxidants obtained through food or supplements have a preventive effect on cardiovascular disease.[12] It is still possible that antioxidants could protect against atherosclerosis if they could be directed to specific sites within the artery wall.

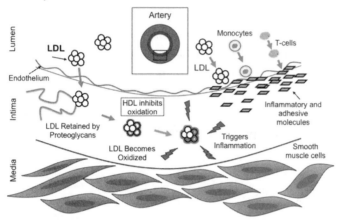

Figure 1.5. The atherosclerotic process starts when LDL particles are retained in the artery wall and trigger an inflammatory and immune response that attracts monocytes and more LDL to the artery. *Figure courtesy of the author.*

Theoretically, preventing the retention of LDL in the arterial wall might be one strategy for inhibiting atherosclerosis. By interfering with the production of apo B in LDL or stopping it from binding to proteoglycans, it might be possible to halt atherosclerosis before it starts. For example, one type of experimental drug, called an antisense inhibitor of apo B, is currently being tested in humans and "turns off" the gene for apo B so that fewer apo B and LDL particles are produced.[13] Another approach involves introducing antibodies to apo B or LDL in order to trigger an immune response, disrupt the molecular interactions that lead to plaque growth, and hopefully protect against atherosclerosis and cardiovascular disease.[14] It may be a while, if ever, before these kinds of experimental therapies gain widespread use, but it is promising that scientists are able to understand the development of atherosclerotic disease at such a basic molecular level.

After the initiation of the atherosclerotic process, cholesterol begins to accumulate within the artery wall (see figure 1.6). The monocytes that have been drawn into the intima are converted to *macrophages*, which are specialized white blood cells capable of consuming other cells or parts of cells. Oxidized or chemically modified LDL is then ingested by the macrophages, which become larger and larger due to the cholesterol carried by LDL. Soon the macrophages become what are known as *foam cells*, stuffed with lipid. This stage of atherosclerosis can be initiated as early as childhood or adolescence and is characterized by the appearance of *fatty streaks*. A fatty streak is a flat, yellowish-white patch made up of foam cells that forms on the inside of an artery but does not block blood flow. Fatty streaks cannot be detected by medical tests, but evidence from autopsies has shown that fatty streaks can develop in children as young as one year of age.[15] They do not necessarily grow in size to become mature atherosclerotic plaques associated with heart disease.

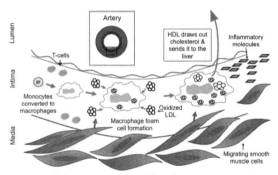

Figure 1.6. Monocytes are converted to macrophages and consume oxidized LDL, while HDL draws cholesterol out of the developing plaque and sends it to the liver. *Figure courtesy of the author.*

At the same time that LDL is deposited into the arterial wall, HDL draws cholesterol out of macrophages through specialized receptors and transports it back to the liver for disposal. This process is called *reverse cholesterol transport* and is believed to be one of the important properties of HDL. HDL may also protect against atherosclerosis by directly combating inflammation and the oxidation of LDL within the arterial wall.[16] In population studies, risk for coronary heart disease decreases by about 2 percent in men and 3 percent in women for each 1 mg/dL increase in HDL cholesterol.[17]

As foam cells in the developing plaque continue to grow, they eventually die, but the lipid they contain accumulates to form a liquid or semi-liquid core. Smooth muscle cells, which normally constitute the middle layer of the arterial wall, begin to proliferate and migrate into the intima, where they contribute to the growth of the maturing plaque. In addition, the connective tissues within the arteries begin to break down. At this stage, which generally occurs during young adulthood and middle age, the atherosclerotic lesion may begin to grow into the lumen (interior of the artery), but it does not produce symptoms. If the plaque continues to grow, its lipid core becomes sealed into the arterial wall by only a thin layer of cells.

If this situation sounds somewhat precarious, that would be a correct assessment. Atherosclerotic plaques are prone to rupture as they grow and begin to protrude into the lumen (see figure 1.7a). Previously, researchers believed that the plaques most prone to rupture were those that caused the largest blockages, or had the greatest degree of *stenosis* (narrowing), within the artery. They now know that *vulnerable plaques* that cause arterial narrowing of 30 to 50 percent but only have a thin layer of fibrous tissue surrounding the lipid core are the most common causes of coronary events (see figure 1.7b).[18] Many people with atherosclerosis have several plaques with less severe narrowing. Plaques that narrow arteries by 70 to 90 percent are relatively less common, but when they do occur, they are highly likely to have adverse consequences (see figure 1.7c).

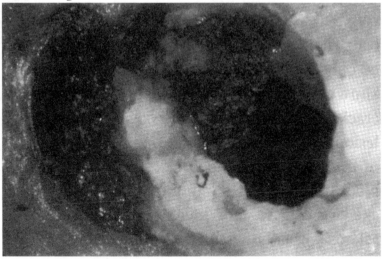

Figure 1.7a. When a plaque ruptures, its contents are exposed to the blood, and it causes a clot to form in the artery. *Figure courtesy of Dr. Michael J. Davies.*

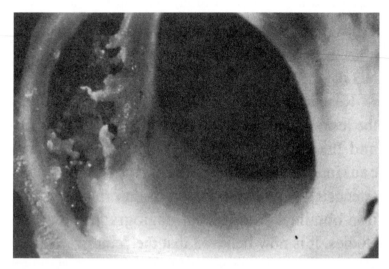

Figure 1.7b. A vulnerable plaque with only a thin layer of cells separating it from the interior of the artery is likely to rupture. *Figure courtesy of Dr. Michael J. Davies.*

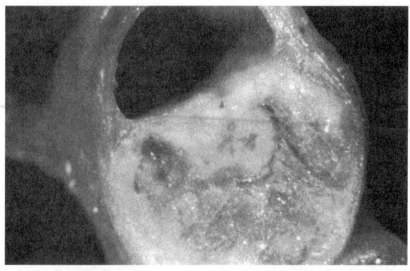

Figure 1.7c. Plaques with severe stenosis are relatively less common. *Figure courtesy of Dr. Michael J. Davies.*

LOWERING LDL-C REDUCES RISK FOR CARDIOVASCULAR DISEASE

LDL-C levels are more closely related to the risk for heart disease than are total cholesterol levels. Numerous studies have shown that high levels of LDL-C are linked to increased risk for heart disease and that reducing LDL-C levels decreases cardiovascular risk. Results from clinical trials conducted over three decades indicate that there is a direct relationship between LDL-C levels and the risk for heart disease (see figure 1.8).[19] For example, an analysis of twenty-six clinical trials with statins, which included over 170,000 participants, found that for each 39 mg/dL (1 mmol/L) reduction in LDL-C, a person's risk for heart disease and stroke decreases by 22 percent.[20] In general, decreases in LDL-C have been shown to lead to fewer heart attacks, reduced angina, fewer hospital procedures to unblock clogged arteries, and fewer deaths due to heart disease. These improved outcomes are observed whether LDL-C reduction is achieved through diet and lifestyle changes alone or with the aid of lipid-lowering drugs.[21]

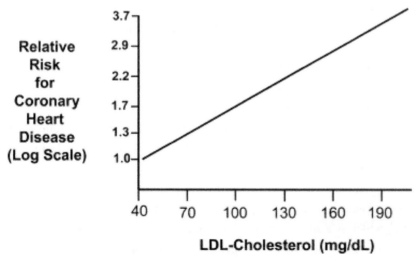

Figure 1.8. There is a direct relationship between LDL-C levels and risk for coronary heart disease. *Figure reprinted from the Journal of the American College of Cardiology, volume 44, issue 3, SM Grundy et al, Implications of Recent Clinical Trials for the National Cholesterol Education Program Adult Treatment Panel III Guidelines, pp. 720–32, © 2004, with permission from Elsevier.*

For individuals with high LDL-C, the first strategy is lifestyle modification, which includes engaging in aerobic exercise, stopping smoking, and eating a healthier diet (see chapter 2 for more on risk factors and prevention). If these measures do not sufficiently reduce LDL-C, a physician may recommend drug therapy based on your estimated risk of developing heart disease within the next ten years. A class of lipid-lowering drug called *statins* has been shown to be the most effective and safest means of reducing LDL-C levels and cardiovascular risk in many different populations. People with an existing history of heart disease have been shown to benefit from LDL-C reduction with statins. Efforts to prevent a recurrent coronary event are called *secondary prevention*. Individuals without heart disease, including people who do not have elevated levels of LDL-C but who may have other cardiovascular risk factors, also experience fewer heart attacks and coronary events the more they lower their LDL-C levels. Efforts to prevent heart disease before it develops and causes symptoms are called *primary prevention*. Trials have shown that both men and women at risk can greatly reduce their chances of ever developing heart disease with preventive treatment with statins (see chapter 2 for more on statins).

For example, one of the authors (AMG) headed a major study in the 1990s called AFCAPS/TexCAPS, which examined approximately 6,600 healthy individuals with average LDL-C levels and no evidence of heart disease.[22] The average LDL-C for the entire group at the start of the study was 150 mg/dL, which was considered normal at the time. The participants also had HDL-C ("good") levels that were below average. After five years, the group treated with the statin drug lovastatin (Mevacor®) had 37 percent fewer incidents of heart attack, unstable angina, and sudden cardiac death compared to the group given a placebo. In other words, 183 people given a placebo had a first major coronary event, as compared to 116 people in the group given lovastatin, which is a highly statistically significant difference. After treatment, the lovastatin group had an average LDL-C of 115 mg/dL. What studies like this illustrate is that in a given population, some people are more likely to have a coronary event than others. Lifestyle and drug interventions to lower LDL-C levels can help to greatly shift the odds in your favor, although there are other factors that can also affect cardiovascular risk.

During the three decades that lipid-lowering trials have been conducted, researchers have not identified a lower level of LDL-C where risk ends. People who are at the highest risk for a coronary event experience the most benefit from reducing their LDL-C. You may have heard research about cholesterol reported in the news. Often these reports are framed as a question: Is lower better? With regards to LDL-C, the "bad" cholesterol, the answer seems to be yes. The lower your levels of LDL-C, the less likely you are to develop atherosclerosis and symptoms of heart disease. If you already have heart disease, reducing your LDL-C to very low levels (<70 mg/dL) can substantially diminish the probability of having another coronary event. In the JUPITER study, discussed below, risk was lowest when LDL-C levels fell to below 50 mg/dL. [23] In addition, studies of different populations show that hunter-gatherers generally had LDL-C levels between 50 and 70 mg/dL and very low incidence of coronary heart disease.[24] As these societies adopted more modern diets and lifestyles, they became more prone to developing CHD, which suggests that very low levels of LDL-C may be ideal in preventing cardiovascular disease in contemporary life. Very low levels of LDL-C, combined with increased levels of HDL-C, may even lead to regression of atherosclerotic plaques (see below).

Several secondary prevention trials conducted after the introduction of statins in 1987 have established that reducing levels of LDL-C improves survival in patients who have already developed CHD. One of the most convincing of these trials was the five-year Heart Protection Study, which included over twenty thousand high-risk individuals with atherosclerotic disease, diabetes, or hypertension (high blood pressure).[25] In the group treated with the statin drug simvastatin (Zocor®), the chances of dying from a coronary event were reduced by approximately 18 percent, and the risk of a heart attack was lowered by at least one-third. Patients experienced benefit with statin treatment regardless of what their LDL-C levels were at the beginning of the trial. The study investigators estimated that treatment with simvastatin for five years would prevent a coronary event in seventy to one hundred people for every one thousand individuals, with longer treatment providing additional benefit. This study included a large number of women, elderly patients, and diabetic patients, and it helped prove that statin therapy is beneficial in these populations.

Since then, a number of secondary prevention studies have investigated whether "lower is better" in patients with CHD. For example, the Treating to New Targets study, for which one of the authors (AMG) served on the steering committee, attempted to reduce LDL-C levels to much less than 100 mg/dL.[26] At the time, patients with a recent heart attack were recommended to have an LDL-C less than 100 mg/dL. In this study, all patients received the statin drug atorvastatin (Lipitor®), but one group (the "intensive" arm) received a higher dose than the other. After approximately five years of treatment, the high-dose group had an average LDL-C of 77 mg/dL, compared to 101 mg/dL in the standard-dose group. A total of 434 patients (8.7 percent) in the high-dose group experienced a major cardiovascular event, compared to 548 patients (10.9 percent) in the standard-dose group, which is a highly statistically significant difference. Trials such as these provided evidence that lowering LDL-C to very low levels is both safe and effective in secondary prevention. As a result, national cholesterol treatment guidelines were changed so that the LDL-C goal for some high-risk patients with CHD was lowered to less than 70 mg/dL.

During the 1980s, there was some concern among researchers that lowering levels of blood cholesterol would also reduce the amount of cholesterol needed by cells, particularly cells in the brain, which could possibly lead to adverse consequences. This theory has been strongly refuted. Reductions in blood cholesterol do not affect the body's proper functioning, and an appropriate balance of cholesterol is maintained throughout the body even as levels decrease in the blood. An analysis of twenty-six major statin trials involving more than 170,000 total participants showed that decreases in blood cholesterol did not increase the risk for cancer or death from non-cardiovascular causes, even at very low LDL-C levels.[27] Furthermore, trials with very strong statins have investigated the effects of reducing LDL-C below 70 mg/dL in patients with and without heart disease, and they consistently show cardiovascular benefit with little to no increase in adverse drug side effects, even at these low levels.

One of these trials, called JUPITER, was completed in 2008 and provides striking evidence that in primary prevention, achieving very low levels of LDL-C can prevent heart attacks and coronary events in healthy patients who already have relatively low LDL-C. This important trial continues to be hotly debated among physicians and cardiovascular researchers, as it reinforces the fact that LDL-C reduction is beneficial but it also suggests that reducing inflammation may be another vital factor to consider.

WHY IS INFLAMMATION IMPORTANT?

Inflammation is the body's natural response to an injury. If you fall and sprain your ankle, the area becomes red and inflamed as blood flow to the area is increased and the body attempts to repair the damaged tissue. However, if inflammation becomes chronic, it can cause damage of its own. Inflammation draws different types of cells to the injured area than are normally present, eventually beginning to change the local environment and its natural balance after a period of time.

Researchers now believe that atherosclerosis is a chronic inflammatory disease. When the arterial wall becomes damaged, either by LDL particles or the effects of diabetes, smoking, or high blood pressure, the result is inflammation, which provides the right environment for an atherosclerotic lesion to grow. Inflammation within blood vessels may also make a plaque more likely to rupture and form a blood clot in a process known as *thrombosis*. The clotting of blood occurs through a rapid series of steps and is affected by the presence or absence of various molecules and cells in the area. When an atherosclerotic plaque is inflamed, it contains high levels of tissue factor, which is the primary molecule responsible for initiating the blood-clotting process. If the plaque is disrupted, or if its edges begin to erode, the insides of the plaque, including the high levels of tissue factor, may quickly become exposed to the surrounding blood, which may have also been altered due to chronic inflammation in the area. The result is thrombosis, or the formation of a blood clot.

C-reactive protein (CRP) is one marker of inflammation that has been consistently linked to increased cardiovascular risk in both men and women. In the JUPITER study, participants were healthy, middle-aged individuals with low LDL-C but elevated levels of CRP.[28] It was the first study to test the hypothesis that statin treatment in individuals with elevated CRP but low LDL-C levels

(<130 mg/dL) would reduce cardiovascular risk. In JUPITER, half of the participants were treated with the statin drug rosuvastatin (Crestor®), and half were
given a placebo. Early on in the trial, it became apparent to the study investigators, which included one of the authors (AMG), that the rosuvastatin group was
doing much better than the group given a placebo and much better than had
been projected based on experience with earlier trials. The study was originally
planned to last five years, but after just two years, it was stopped early because
it was clear that drug treatment was superior to placebo in this population of
individuals. If the trial had continued for the full five years, it would likely have
shown even greater benefit with drug treatment, but the way that clinical trials
are designed made it more practical to terminate it early.

   After two years, the group treated with rosuvastatin had reduced their
LDL-C by 50 percent and their CRP levels by 37 percent. These healthy
individuals already had low levels of LDL-C to begin with (median 108 mg/
dL), and LDL-C was further decreased to a median of 55 mg/dL. The results
showed that treatment with rosuvastatin led to half as many heart attacks
and strokes compared to treatment with a placebo. It was estimated that only
twenty-five people needed to be treated with rosuvastatin for five years to
prevent one major coronary event, which represents an extremely good success
rate. In addition, the risk of death from any cause was found to be 20 percent
less for individuals in the rosuvastatin group compared to those in the placebo
group. The study participants who experienced the greatest reductions in cardiovascular risk were those who achieved the lowest levels of both LDL-C
and CRP by the end of the study.[29] These results suggest that reducing both
LDL-C and CRP may confer the greatest benefit in primary prevention, rather
than simply targeting LDL-C alone.

   CRP is most likely a sign of the inflammation that accompanies atherosclerosis, rather than something that directly causes atherosclerosis itself.
Statins other than rosuvastatin have been shown to reduce levels of CRP, and it
is hypothesized that in addition to reducing LDL-C, statins reduce inflammation more generally and, thus, measures of CRP. In other words, it is important to reduce inflammation in order to decrease cardiovascular risk, and CRP
is one of the most reliable markers of the inflammation associated with atherosclerosis. It may be the case that "lower is better" for both LDL-C and CRP.

Current guidelines for physicians do not yet recommend routine screening for CRP, although they do suggest that testing for CRP may be useful in certain cases where it is unclear whether or not the patient should begin lipid-lowering drug therapy. You may want to consider asking your doctor about testing for CRP levels. CRP is measured with an inexpensive blood test that can be ordered at the same time that your cholesterol levels are being measured. In the JUPITER trial, participants initially had CRP levels greater than 2 mg/L, which is considered high, and individuals whose CRP reached levels less than 1 mg/L by the end of the trial experienced the best results. If your levels are elevated, there are several ways to lower your CRP in addition to statin therapy.

Often people with elevated levels of CRP also have other risk factors for heart disease, such as obesity and a sedentary lifestyle. Like atherosclerosis, obesity is believed to produce a state of chronic, low-grade inflammation within the body's tissues. In obese individuals, fat cells release an abundance of hormones and inflammatory molecules, which then attract macrophages in a process very similar to atherosclerosis.[30] The resulting inflammatory environment may help explain why obese individuals are at higher risk for developing conditions such as cardiovascular disease and diabetes. Losing weight, in addition to increasing exercise and stopping smoking, can help reduce elevated levels of CRP.

Aspirin has long been recommended for the prevention of heart attacks, particularly in men. It is now recognized that aspirin can also help to prevent strokes in older women.[31] Previously, it was thought that aspirin worked to prevent heart attacks by acting as a blood thinner, thereby decreasing the likelihood that clots would form. It now appears that aspirin also reduces inflammation within blood vessels, which decreases the odds that a plaque will rupture in the first place to form a blood clot. Although aspirin does not seem to reduce CRP levels on its own, it is hypothesized that aspirin may be especially helpful in preventing heart attacks in individuals who have elevated levels of CRP.[32]

Inflammation is currently a hot area of cardiovascular research. Scientists and physicians are still working to understand the complex relationship between inflammation, atherosclerosis, and heart disease. Trials are underway to test whether anti-inflammatory drugs may be beneficial in decreasing cardiovascular events. What is clear now is that strategies to reduce inflammation throughout the body, including weight loss, quitting smoking, increased exercise, aspirin, and statins, are likely to improve your chances of never developing symptoms of heart disease.

REVERSING THE ATHEROSCLEROTIC PROCESS

The progression of atherosclerosis is not always relentless, as was previously thought. With aggressive lifestyle changes and appropriate drug therapy, atherosclerosis can be stopped and, at times, even reversed. Beginning in the late 1980s, clinical trials using various imaging techniques, which allow physicians to view plaque growth within the arteries, have demonstrated that it is possible to halt atherosclerotic progression and, in some cases, even induce *regression* (decrease in size) of plaques. In general, these studies have demonstrated that even relatively small changes in arterial blockage can result in unexpectedly large reductions in coronary events.

Recent studies have utilized sophisticated imaging techniques, including intravascular ultrasound (IVUS), electron-beam computed tomography (EBCT), and high-resolution magnetic resonance imaging (MRI) (see chapter 3 for more on diagnostic tests). IVUS is an invasive procedure that provides a cross-sectional image of the interior of a blood vessel, including the size and dimensions of plaques. EBCT scans show the presence of calcium deposits in the arteries surrounding the heart, which can be an early sign of heart disease before symptoms begin to develop. Cardiac MRIs can provide still and moving images of the heart and large arteries.

Advances in imaging have yielded valuable data on the progression of atherosclerosis and help document the effects of different drugs on the size and shape of atherosclerotic plaques. However, the use of imaging in clinical trials remains somewhat controversial among researchers. It is well established that changes in LDL-C levels are linked to improved outcomes, such as fewer heart attacks and improved life expectancy. There is not the same level of evidence for imaging yet, so it is not entirely clear what effect decreases in plaque size, for example, would have on the risk for heart attack, although such changes are likely to be beneficial.

Some studies using high-resolution MRI suggest that statin therapy may help to stabilize atherosclerotic plaques so they are less prone to rupture. These studies show that drug treatment with statins may change the composition or size of plaques, but that it does not always decrease the degree of blockage within the artery. Other trials have investigated the effects of drugs in patients already taking statins. Once a patient has been on statin therapy for several years, it may be difficult to show further beneficial effects with other drugs since the statin will already have reduced the lipid content of plaques.

Studies incorporating IVUS provide the strongest evidence that statins can slow or reverse the progression of atherosclerosis within the vessel wall. The ASTEROID trial, published in 2006, was one of the first trials to demonstrate either regression or a stop in progression.[33] It included 349 individuals with coronary atherosclerosis who received a high dose of rosuvastatin for two years. At the end of the study, these individuals had reduced their LDL-C by 53 percent to a mean of 61 mg/dL, and they had increased their HDL-C by 15 percent. According to three different measurements obtained with IVUS, the volume of their plaques decreased in size by approximately 7 percent. This study confirmed that reducing LDL-C to very low levels can actually reverse atherosclerosis, which should be heartening news for people who may have already developed heart disease or who have evidence of atherosclerotic plaques.

A subsequent analysis combined data from ASTEROID and three other similar IVUS trials, and it included 1,455 patients with coronary artery disease who were treated with statins for eighteen to twenty-four months.[34] This analysis found that substantial atherosclerotic regression (≥ 5 percent reduction in plaque volume) was most likely to occur in patients who had achieved LDL-C levels below 87.5 mg/dL combined with an increase in HDL-C greater than 7.5 percent. This study suggests that reducing LDL-C to very low levels, combined with an increase in HDL-C, may be the best way to reduce cardiovascular risk.

These imaging studies confirm that halting the spread of atherosclerosis is not beyond your control. As we will see in the next chapter, the chances of developing cardiovascular disease are affected by many risk factors. However, taking preventive measures aimed at controlling lipid levels and blood pressure, stopping smoking, increasing physical activity, maintaining a healthy weight, and consuming a balanced diet can literally save your life. In the twenty-first century, physicians know more about atherosclerosis, its consequences, and its prevention than ever before. Now let's see what concrete steps you can take to protect yourself from heart disease.

CHAPTER 2

RISK FACTORS AND PREVENTION IN THE 21st CENTURY

U nderstanding how atherosclerosis develops and leads to coronary heart disease is the first step in prevention. The second is understanding how various risk factors promote atherosclerosis and the chances of having a coronary event or stroke so that you can address and change your risk factors before heart disease or other forms of atherosclerotic vascular disease develop. If you already have atherosclerotic disease, controlling your risk factors is key to decreasing symptoms and preventing future events. This chapter describes the most important risk factors for heart disease and other forms of atherosclerotic vascular disease, as well as the recommended strategies for improving and controlling them.

A *risk factor* is defined as any trait or habit that helps predict the probability that a person will develop a particular disease. Risk factors can be genetic or environmental; some are related to lifestyle. Multiple risk factors greatly increase the risk for cardiovascular disease and have a multiplicative, rather than simply an additive, effect on risk. For example, the INTERHEART study examined over fifteen thousand cases of heart attacks in fifty-two countries and found that nine potentially modifiable risk factors accounted for over 90 percent of the risk for heart attacks in men and women of all ethnicities.[1] The nine risk factors were smoking, lipids, high blood pressure, diabetes, obesity, psychosocial factors (stress), diet, alcohol consumption, and physical inactivity. Having one of the risk factors, such as diabetes, could as much as triple the risk for heart attack, but having all nine of the risk factors increased the likelihood of having a heart attack by a factor of 129. Fortunately, these nine risk factors can all be modified by diet and lifestyle, as well as by medication if necessary. Many of the fifteen thousand heart attacks included in the study thus might have been prevented.

Risk factor modification is proven to work. Even though cardiovascular disease remains the leading cause of death in the United States, cardiovascular mortality rates have been declining. From 1997 to 2007, deaths from cardiovascular disease decreased by 28 percent.[2] Approximately half of the decrease in mortality over the past several decades is believed to be due to improved control of risk factors, such as cholesterol, blood pressure, smoking, and physical inactivity.[3] The other half is attributed to improvements in medical and surgical procedures to treat heart disease. These results should be encouraging: efforts at prevention are working, while existing treatments for heart disease are helping to extend life. The goal for you now is to focus on prevention and avoid the need for more serious treatments. At stake is not just length of life, but quality of life.

ESTIMATING RISK

In the United States, the National Cholesterol Education Program (NCEP), which is sponsored by the National Institutes of Health, issues guidelines for physicians about identifying and treating high cholesterol in order to reduce the risk for heart disease across the population. These guidelines are endorsed by the American Heart Association (AHA) and many other professional organizations. They establish target levels for one of the major risk factors for heart disease: high cholesterol and, more specifically, LDL-C.

Controlling LDL-C ("bad" cholesterol) has been shown in numerous studies involving many different groups of people to have the single greatest effect in reducing cardiovascular risk. If a person has high LDL-C, the guidelines set an appropriate LDL-C target based on whether the patient already has heart disease, other forms of atherosclerotic disease, diabetes, or any of the other major risk factors. These major risk factors include cigarette smoking, hypertension (high blood pressure), low HDL-C ("good" cholesterol), family history of premature coronary heart disease, male gender, and age (see table 2.1). Risk factors determined by lifestyle, including obesity, physical inactivity, and diet, are also important in the development of heart disease, as are new or "emerging" risk factors, such as those related to inflammation. Trying to improve all of these risk factors will help reduce your risk of developing heart disease as well as other forms of atherosclerotic vascular disease, such as stroke or peripheral artery disease.

Table 2.1. Major Risk Factors for Coronary Heart Disease in Addition to LDL-C[4]

Risk Factor	Definition
Cigarette smoking	Any
High blood pressure	BP ≥ 140/90 mm Hg; or on blood pressure medication
Low HDL-C*	< 40 mg/dL
Family history of premature CHD	CHD in male first-degree relative < 55 years; CHD in female first-degree relative < 65 years
Age	men ≥ 45 years; women ≥ 55 years

* HDL-C ≥ 60 mg/dL is a "negative" risk factor that removes 1 risk factor from the total count.

If you have two or more major risk factors, your doctor may estimate your risk of developing a heart attack within the next ten years using a calculation called the Framingham risk score. This formula is based on data obtained from an ongoing, landmark study called the Framingham Heart Study, which is following a large group of people from Framingham, Massachusetts, and their descendants, in order to determine what risk factors predispose to heart disease. An easy-to-use version of the calculator is available online at http://hp2010.nhlbihin.net/atpiii/calculator.asp.

It is important to remember that the Framingham score provides an estimate of risk and primarily helps doctors determine how low your LDL-C should be based on your existing risk factors. A low score does not necessarily mean that you are safe from heart disease, and a high score does not mean that you will definitely have a heart attack. For example, in the JUPITER study, most of the cardiovascular events occurred in people with below average risk. According to their Framingham score, these individuals only had an estimated 5 to 10 percent chance of having a heart attack within the next ten years, yet they still happened to suffer a coronary event during the two-year study period.[5] If you do have a high score, don't despair. There is a lot you can do to reduce your odds for developing heart disease. If you have a low score, you should also seriously consider the steps you can take to protect yourself further against heart disease.

Most likely, you are familiar with many of these preventive measures already: don't smoke, exercise more, eat healthy, lose weight if needed, and take the medications your doctor prescribes. What this chapter will explain is the scientific and medical rationale behind these recommendations so that you understand why and how the choices that you make can slow, or even reverse, the atherosclerotic process. Furthermore, you'll learn how many risk factors are interrelated and why multiple risk factors tend to cluster in the same individual. This knowledge is key to making strategic lifestyle choices that will benefit your cardiovascular system on many different levels. In addition, we describe some of the kinds of medications your doctor might prescribe in order to decrease your risk factors.

NON-MODIFIABLE RISK FACTORS

Let's begin with the risk factors that cannot be modified. Keep in mind that although these factors cannot be changed, it is still possible to counteract their effects, in part by improving the risk factors that can be controlled.

Personal History of Coronary Heart Disease

If you already have CHD or another form of atherosclerotic vascular disease, including a history of angina, heart attack, stroke, peripheral artery disease, abdominal aortic aneurysm, or carotid artery disease, you are at very high risk for a future coronary event. American Heart Association statistics show that within five years of a first heart attack, 15 percent of men and 22 percent of women aged 45–64 will suffer another heart attack, and 2 percent of men and 6 percent of women will have a stroke.[6] One of the reasons for this increased risk should be readily apparent: once atherosclerosis has developed in an artery to the point that you experience symptoms or a coronary event, it is likely to have also affected blood flow in other arteries throughout the body. If you survive a heart attack and are treated with a stent or bypass surgery, these procedures restore blood flow only through the most severely blocked arteries (see chapter 5 for more on treatments for coronary heart disease). Without intensive lifestyle changes and drug therapies, atherosclerosis may continue to progress in other arteries, possibly leading to a subsequent coronary event. In addition, heart attacks damage the heart muscle, decreasing its efficiency in pumping blood throughout the body and increasing the likelihood of heart failure, sudden cardiac death, and other conditions.

In people with CHD, the physician's goal is called secondary prevention, or preventing a recurrent coronary event. The first priority is to lower LDL-C levels at least below 100 mg/dL (milligrams per deciliter of blood) and preferably below 70 mg/dL. Clinical research studies have shown that individuals with a history of coronary heart disease fare much better after lowering their blood cholesterol levels. In an important study called 4S, which was conducted in men and women with a history of angina or heart attack, cholesterol lowering with the statin drug simvastatin (Zocor®) reduced both the risk for a future coronary event and the risk for death by about one-third over a period of five years.[7] People with coronary heart disease should not underestimate the benefit of keeping cholesterol levels as low as possible. Even in individuals with average cholesterol levels who have suffered a heart attack, cholesterol lowering with statins has been shown to reduce the risk of a recurrent event by approximately 20 to 25 percent.[8]

If you have a history of coronary heart disease, focus on lowering cholesterol levels through diet, exercise, and appropriate drug therapy in order to shift the odds in your favor. Pay increased attention to the other modifiable risk factors discussed later in this chapter.

Age

Risk for atherosclerotic disease increases with the aging process, in part because other risk factors such as blood pressure, cholesterol, and body weight tend to increase with age. The adverse effects of risk factors also accumulate over a lifetime so that a person who has had high cholesterol for fifty years, for example, is likely to have sustained more total damage to his arteries than someone in his twenties. For this reason, efforts to prevent heart disease by paying attention to cardiovascular risk factors, especially LDL-C levels, should begin early in life. Human infants are born with LDL-C levels around 50 mg/dL. Studies have shown that individuals who have low levels of LDL-C during childhood and young adulthood, whether due to genetic factors or lifestyle, are less likely to develop atherosclerosis and heart disease as they age. For example, one study found that African Americans with a genetic variant that causes LDL-C levels that are on average 28 percent lower than those found in the general population have an 88 percent decreased risk for heart disease.[9] Individuals without such genetic variants could similarly benefit from maintaining low LDL-C levels across their life span.

Men older than forty-five years and women older than fifty-five years are at increased risk for cardiovascular disease compared to younger individuals. Coronary events such as heart attack or the need for bypass surgery are fairly uncommon in men until they reach their midforties and in women before their midfifties. In men aged thirty-five to forty-four, the average annual rate for a first cardiovascular event is 3 in 1,000.[10] This rate increases steadily with age and, in men ages eighty-five to ninety-four years, is 74 in 1,000. Rates are similar for women, although on average there tends to be a ten-year delay in the occurrence of a first cardiovascular event in women who are not diabetic and who do not smoke. This delay occurs because estrogen levels in premenopausal women have a protective effect in the development of heart disease.

The major risk factors for coronary heart disease and other atherosclerotic diseases are still very important in older adults. Studies with statins show that younger and older adults both experience similar reductions in the risk for cardiovascular events with cholesterol-lowering therapy.[11] Statin therapy is safe in elderly individuals, although older adults may be more prone to side effects and may require lower drug dosages. Since individuals older than sixty-five years of age are at the highest risk for heart disease, this group has the most to gain from risk factor intervention.

Sex

Heart disease is the leading cause of death for both men and women, although it affects women differently. As discussed above, men tend to develop heart disease about ten years earlier than women. Coronary heart disease is much less common in premenopausal women than in men of the same age. The hormones that regulate the menstrual cycle, especially estrogen, appear to protect most women (although not diabetic women) against coronary heart disease during their reproductive years. In the diabetic woman, there may be some protection by estrogen, but the relative risk for heart disease is increased to approximately that of a man her same age due to the effects of diabetes. Once a woman goes through menopause, her coronary heart disease risk rises dramatically, although men are still at comparatively higher risk.

Following menopause, the increase in coronary heart disease incidence appears to be due at least partially to changes in lipid levels that make a woman more susceptible to developing atherosclerosis. Before women reach menopause, they tend to have lower LDL ("bad") cholesterol and higher HDL ("good") cholesterol than men of approximately the same age. Starting at menopause, women's LDL-C levels begin to rise rapidly with increasing age, until the levels may actually be higher than LDL-C levels in men. Women's HDL-C levels may decrease moderately at menopause, although they do ordinarily remain higher than men's HDL-C levels from the time of puberty on, throughout the life span. There is little difference in triglyceride levels between boys and girls at puberty. Triglyceride levels increase gradually in both men and women after puberty, although they increase at a slower pace in women. In middle age, when triglyceride levels may actually decrease in men, they continue to increase gradually in women so that by age seventy, average triglyceride levels in women are equal to those of men.

Oral estrogen in postmenopausal women, or hormone replacement therapy (HRT), had been shown to reduce LDL-C to premenopausal levels and to increase HDL-C. During the 1990s, studies suggested that HRT might protect against women's increased risk for heart disease following menopause. Nevertheless, in 2002 the results of a large study involving 160,000 women, called the Women's Health Initiative, provided conclusive evidence that oral estrogen does not reduce the risk for heart attack and that it in fact increases the risk for stroke and blood clots.[12] As a result, HRT is not recommended for the prevention of heart disease or stroke. Short-term use may be appropriate for the treatment of menopausal symptoms, but long-term use is discouraged because it may increase risk for heart disease, stroke, and breast cancer. Women should talk with their physicians about the potential benefits and risks of hormone therapy in the context of their own medical histories and that of their immediate family members.

In recent years there have been efforts to increase awareness in women of their risk for heart disease, such as the American Heart Association's Go Red™ for Women movement. Many women may not realize that heart disease is the leading cause of death for women and may think of it as a disease primarily affecting older men. This lack of awareness may prevent women from seeking prompt medical attention for potential heart problems. Women are more likely than men to experience periodic episodes of angina, or chest pain, as the first symptom of coronary heart disease (see chapter 4 for more on angina). However, women are also more likely to ignore their chest pain or other heart disease symptoms, to attribute their symptoms to another cause such as indigestion or a pulled muscle, and to postpone getting treatment even if they do suspect a problem.

Coronary heart disease represents a very real threat to women. One of the most important things a woman can do is to become aware of her own cardiovascular risk factors. Women should also be sure that their risk for heart disease is evaluated by their physician as part of their regular health care regimen, and they should familiarize themselves with the early symptoms of coronary heart disease and with the symptoms of angina in particular. For both women and men, controlling risk factors by leading a healthy lifestyle is central to reducing the risk for coronary heart disease.

Family History of Premature Coronary Heart Disease

Coronary heart disease tends to cluster in families, and a family history of premature heart disease greatly increases cardiovascular risk. The NCEP defines a family history of heart disease as having a father, brother, or son who suffered a heart attack or sudden coronary death before age fifty-five, or having a mother, sister, or daughter who had a heart attack or sudden coronary death before age sixty-five. If you are at increased risk for heart disease because of your family history, focus on lifestyle changes to reduce your overall risk. Also, try to help family members make lifestyle changes that will reduce their risk for heart disease.

MODIFIABLE RISK FACTORS

Modifiable risk factors are affected primarily by dietary and lifestyle choices. It is important that children learn and adhere to healthy habits throughout their lifetimes. Atherosclerosis begins to develop at an early age, even if the disease does not become symptomatic until years later. For example, in 1953 scientists performed autopsies on two thousand American soldiers who had died in the Korean War.[13] More than three-quarters of these young, healthy soldiers, who were on average aged twenty-two years, had "fatty streaks," or the beginnings of atherosclerotic plaques, within their coronary arteries. Fatty streaks generally begin to develop during the teenage years, although they have even been found in infants. Unhealthy, sedentary lifestyles can accelerate the development of full-blown atherosclerotic disease, so it is essential that you pay careful attention to the modifiable risk factors at all stages of life. Maintaining a low LDL-C level throughout your life span is likely to have a far greater impact on decreasing your risk for heart disease than waiting until you are middle-aged. However, if you do not follow a healthy lifestyle now, it is never too late to make a change.

Many modifiable risk factors are interrelated, so making a change in one risk factor can also have beneficial effects on others. For example, lowering fat intake can improve your blood cholesterol levels, and it can also help with weight loss and, subsequently, blood pressure control. All of these changes have a cumulative effect on cardiovascular risk reduction.

Lipids

Lipid disorders in general are referred to by physicians as *dyslipidemia* and can take several common forms. High levels of total cholesterol or LDL-C are called *hypercholesterolemia*.[14] Elevated triglycerides are called *hypertriglyceridemia* and can occur in isolation or along with low levels of HDL-C. The combination of high triglycerides, low HDL-C, and small dense LDL particles, which is common in individuals with diabetes or the metabolic syndrome (see the sections in this chapter on diabetes and obesity), is referred to as the *lipid triad* or *atherogenic dyslipidemia*. There are also a number of rare hereditary conditions that can cause very abnormal lipid levels. Some people may be genetically predisposed to developing a few more common forms of lipid disorders, particularly if they have close family members with dyslipidemia.

All adults should have their cholesterol levels measured every five years, beginning at age twenty. A sample of blood is usually obtained from a vein in the arm, or a few drops are drawn from a pinprick to the finger. Children and adolescents over the age of two who have a family history of premature CHD or high cholesterol, unknown family history, or other risk factors for heart disease, such as smoking, diabetes, high blood pressure, obesity, or physical inactivity, should also have their lipid levels checked. Do not change what you typically eat or drink before having your lipid levels measured.

A full lipid profile determines levels of total blood cholesterol, HDL-C, LDL-C, and triglycerides and can be obtained in a fasting or non-fasting state, although fasting is preferable. Triglyceride measurements are only accurate after fasting. If you are asked to fast, do not eat or drink anything except water for twelve hours before the test. As mentioned previously, in the United States, lipid levels are generally reported in milligrams per deciliter of blood (mg/dL). They may also be reported in the metric units of millimoles per liter (mmol/L). To convert total cholesterol, LDL-C, or HDL-C values from mmol/L to mg/dL, multiply by 38.7. To convert triglyceride values from mmol/L to mg/dL, multiply by 88.6.

Classifications of total cholesterol, LDL-C, HDL-C, and triglyceride levels for adults are given in table 2.2. Some researchers believe that other lipid measures are more closely related to the risk for atherosclerosis and heart disease than LDL-C. Some of these alternative measures include the level of apolipo-protein B (a primary component of LDL, IDL, and VLDL), the level of non-HDL-C (which can be calculated by subtracting the HDL-C level from the total cholesterol level), and numbers of LDL or HDL particles (the standard lipid profile measures the amount of cholesterol contained within LDL and HDL particles, not the number of individual particles). While these other measures can sometimes help physicians decide how to treat a particular patient, most doctors rely primarily on levels of LDL-C to guide treatment decisions.

Table 2.2. Classification of LDL-C, Total Cholesterol, HDL-C, and Triglyceride Levels (mg/dL) for Adults[15]

LDL-C		Total Cholesterol		HDL-C		Triglycerides	
< 100	Optimal	< 200	Desirable	< 40	Low	< 150	Normal
100–129	Near or above optimal	200–239	Borderline high	≥ 60	High (desirable)	150–199	Borderline high
130–159	Borderline high	≥ 240	High			200–499	High
160–189	High					≥ 500	Very high
≥ 190	Very high						

Total Cholesterol

Total cholesterol measures all of the cholesterol and triglycerides in the blood, including both LDL-C ("bad") and HDL-C ("good"). Any food of animal origin, including meat, seafood, poultry, and dairy products, contains cholesterol. Egg yolks and organ meat are especially rich sources of dietary cholesterol. However, levels of total cholesterol and LDL-C in the blood become elevated mostly due to excess consumption of saturated fat, usually obtained as animal fat but also found in fried foods and baked goods. Dietary cholesterol can increase total cholesterol in some individuals, but saturated fat is primarily responsible. According to a survey conducted by the National Center for Health Statistics/Centers for Disease Control and Prevention (NCHS/CDC), approximately 15 percent of the US population has high total cholesterol, with levels of 240 mg/dL or higher.[16]

LDL Cholesterol

Measures of LDL-C are more closely linked to the risk for coronary heart disease than measures of total cholesterol. According to the American Heart Association, the mean LDL-C for American adults is 115 mg/dL.[17] Elevated LDL-C in our society commonly results from eating too much dietary fat, especially saturated fat from animal sources. People who follow a vegetarian diet often consume less saturated fat and typically have lower LDL-C levels and decreased rates of coronary heart disease compared to nonvegetarians. Some diseases, such as hypothyroidism and chronic kidney disease, can also elevate LDL-C. Some rare genetic disorders can result in extremely high levels of LDL-C. Many people can have a genetic predisposition to high cholesterol, although in most cases, lifestyle factors such as diet and physical activity determine whether the person will actually develop high cholesterol. For most people, LDL-C is a risk factor well within their control.

If the results from your lipid profile are suboptimal, the first target of lifestyle and drug therapy is always LDL-C. Unless your levels are very high to start or if you have already experienced a cardiovascular event, your physician will probably advise you to try lowering LDL-C through diet and exercise first (see the sections in this chapter on diet and exercise). If these measures are not sufficient, your physician may decide to prescribe lipid-lowering drugs. Doctors set target LDL-C levels based on your number of existing risk factors and your Framingham risk score (see table 2.3). If you have multiple risk factors or have diagnosed heart disease, you will have a lower LDL-C target than if you have none of the major risk factors. In our opinion, even people who are at low risk for heart disease should strive to keep their LDL-C under 130 mg/dL, and preferably under 100 mg/dL if possible, by maintaining a healthy, active lifestyle. Not only will such preventive measures keep your heart strong and your arteries clean, but your overall health, well-being, and quality of life will also benefit.

Table 2.3. LDL-C Goals According to Categories of Risk[18]

Risk Category	LDL-C Goal (mg/dL)
High risk: CHD and CHD-risk equivalents (Clinical atherosclerotic disease, diabetes, 10-yr. CHD risk > 20 %)	< 100
Very high risk	Optional goal of < 70
Moderately high risk: ≥ 2 risk factors (10-yr. risk 10–20 %)	< 130 (Optional goal of < 100)
Moderate risk: ≥ 2 risk factors (10-yr. risk < 10 %)	< 130
Low risk: ≤ 1 risk factor	< 160

Small Dense LDL

A subclass of LDL particles termed small dense LDL may be particularly likely to lead to atherosclerosis. The presence of small dense LDL indicates increased risk for coronary heart disease, particularly in women.[19] Some people may be genetically predisposed to developing small dense LDL particles. These LDL particles have a higher proportion of protein than normal LDL particles, which makes them smaller and denser. Small dense LDL particles may be more susceptible to oxidation, which may make it easier for them to penetrate the arterial wall during the atherosclerotic process. In addition, their smaller size may make it easier for them to be transported by other molecules into the arterial wall. Small dense LDL particles often occur in conjunction with low HDL-C and high triglycerides, a combination associated with especially increased risk and referred to as the lipid triad or atherogenic dyslipidemia. The lipid triad is commonly found in people with diabetes or the metabolic syndrome (see the sections in this chapter on diabetes and obesity). Increased physical activity and weight loss may help normalize LDL particle size.

Some doctors may choose to measure LDL particle size, but they generally do not do so routinely. Specialized blood tests can be ordered to determine LDL particle size, but they are generally expensive and are not always covered by insurance. Measurements, which are not well standardized, can be made by analyzing the magnetic properties of the particles, by using electrical fields to determine their size, or by separating them using an ultracentrifuge (a machine that spins very quickly). Measures of low HDL-C and high triglycerides, which are part of the standard lipid profile, can often help doctors predict whether a patient is likely to have small dense LDL. Tests for LDL particle size may be helpful in people with a family history of premature CHD who may have possibly inherited small dense LDL as a risk factor. They may also be ordered to help explain why a person with CHD may have developed heart disease if she does not have other risk factors or to determine whether more than one kind of lipid-modifying drug treatment might be necessary in high-risk patients. If small dense LDL particles are found to be elevated, efforts at lifestyle modification should be intensified. Your physician will also determine whether treatment with multiple lipid-modifying drugs may be appropriate to address the various aspects of atherogenic dyslipidemia.

Lipoprotein(a)

Lipoprotein(a), abbreviated as Lp(a) and referred to as "lipoprotein little a" or "Lp little a," is identical to an LDL particle except for the addition of a protein called apolipoprotein(a), or apo(a) ("apo little a"). Apo(a) resembles *plasminogen*, which is a substance important to preventing blood clots. High levels of Lp(a) are linked to increased risk for heart disease. Standard lipid-lowering therapies, including diet and drugs, generally have little effect on Lp(a) levels. Nicotinic acid is the only approved lipid-lowering drug that lowers Lp(a), but it is unclear whether this helps reduce cardiovascular risk. Since the apo(a) molecule associated with Lp(a) resembles plasminogen, it is thought that Lp(a) promotes thrombosis (the formation of blood clots) by interfering with plasminogen's natural activity.

Lp(a) is considered an emerging risk factor. Some physicians may choose to measure your Lp(a) level if they are trying to determine an appropriate LDL-C target based on your major risk factors. Blood samples will need to be sent to specialized laboratories since there are several methods for measuring Lp(a) and they are not standardized for routine use. Since Lp(a) is often produced in different sizes within the same person, the test that is ordered should take into account all of the different Lp(a) varieties. Generally, Lp(a) tests are reserved for patients who have a strong family history of CHD or who might have high cholesterol due to genetic causes. If your levels of Lp(a) are elevated, your doctor may decide to classify you as being at higher risk and to intensify lipid-lowering treatment to a lower LDL-C target.

HDL Cholesterol

HDL transports cholesterol away from growing atherosclerotic lesions. Elevated levels of HDL-C are strongly linked to decreased cardiovascular risk. A low HDL-C, which is defined as less than 40 mg/dL, is a major risk factor for heart disease. A high HDL-C, or a level greater than 60 mg/dL, is considered a "negative" risk factor. If you are a sixty-year-old woman and have a family history of premature CHD, for example, you would have two major risk factors (age and family history). However, if you had those risk factors plus an HDL-C level greater than 60 mg/dL, you would be considered as having just one major risk factor because the protective effects of HDL allow doctors to subtract one risk factor from the total. The guidelines do not set specific goals for increasing HDL-C levels.

Women typically have higher HDL-C levels than men. Low HDL-C levels often result from physical inactivity, obesity, or smoking. Lifestyle measures that raise HDL-C include aerobic exercise, stopping smoking, weight loss, moderate alcohol consumption (up to two drinks per day for men and one drink per day for women), and increased intake of omega-3 fatty acids, which are found primarily in fish. A low HDL-C level often occurs along with high levels of triglyceride.

HDL contains a protein called apolipoprotein A-I (apo A-I), which allows HDL to bind to special receptors (molecules found on the surface of cells that process chemical signals from other cells) that aid in transporting cholesterol out of growing plaques. Some researchers believe that the ratio of apolipoprotein B (a protein contained in LDL, IDL, and VLDL) to apo A-I is useful in estimating a person's risk for heart disease (apo B/apo A-I). Others prefer the ratio of total cholesterol to HDL-C (TC/HDL-C). These ratios may help guide physicians in making treatment decisions, but the primary goal is always to optimize LDL-C levels first. In addition to the lifestyle measures mentioned above, treatment with nicotinic acid (see the section in this chapter on nicotinic acid) is the most effective at raising HDL-C levels.

Triglycerides and Non-HDL Cholesterol

Triglycerides are used by the body for energy and are carried in VLDL, IDL, and chylomicrons. While elevated levels of VLDL and IDL are associated with increased risk for atherosclerotic disease, elevations of chylomicrons are not. However, partially digested chylomicrons and VLDL, called chylomicron remnants and VLDL remnants, do appear to accelerate atherosclerosis. If blood tests are performed without fasting, they will detect the triglycerides carried by chylomicrons and remnant lipoproteins. Lipid profiles obtained after fasting only count the triglycerides contained in VLDL and IDL and are therefore more accurate.

Elevated triglyceride levels often occur in people who also have low HDL-C or who are obese. Since these risk factors often cluster together, it is currently unclear what effect high triglycerides have on cardiovascular risk independent of these other variables. However, elevated triglycerides are definitely associated with increased cardiovascular risk—and people with elevated triglycerides, low HDL-C, and/or obesity are at even higher risk. Levels less than 150 mg/dL are considered normal. Elevated triglyceride levels may be more associated with increased risk in women than in men.

Hypertriglyceridemia can result from diets high in carbohydrates (more than 60 percent of calories) and saturated fat. As mentioned above, individuals who are obese, overweight, or physically inactive often have high triglycerides. Triglycerides can also become elevated due to excess alcohol consumption and cigarette smoking, diabetes and kidney disease, certain drugs (corticosteroids, estrogens, retinoids, and beta-blockers), and very rare genetic disorders. Very high triglyceride levels (above 1,000 mg/dL) increase the risk for *pancreatitis*, a potentially life-threatening inflammation of the pancreas, and should be treated with drugs immediately.

Non-HDL-C is a relatively new measure of "bad" cholesterol that may be used, particularly in patients with high triglycerides. Non-HDL-C includes remnant lipoproteins, VLDL, IDL, and LDL and can be calculated by subtracting the HDL-C level from the total cholesterol level. If you have high triglycerides (but not high enough to increase risk for pancreatitis), your doctor will first treat your LDL-C if necessary, followed by your non-HDL-C.

Non-HDL-C is thus a secondary target of lipid-lowering therapy in patients with high triglycerides. Non-HDL-C can be reduced through weight loss and increased physical activity, as well as by drugs that specifically reduce levels of triglyceride-rich lipoproteins. Isolated high triglycerides can be treated with prescription-strength omega-3 fatty acids. High triglycerides in combination with low HDL-C may require treatment with nicotinic acid or fibrates. Statins also moderately reduce triglycerides (see the section in this chapter on statins).

Medications for Lipid Disorders

If you have a suboptimal lipid profile, you should try first to decrease saturated fat consumption, exercise more, and lose weight if necessary. If these measures are not sufficient, your physician may prescribe a lipid-lowering drug. These drugs may also help to raise your HDL-C level. Lipid-lowering drugs are not a replacement for making lifestyle changes. If your physician recommends that you begin lipid-lowering medication, you will still need to maintain your lifestyle efforts. Continuing to eat a diet high in saturated fat and cholesterol will make the drug work less effectively. In addition, improving your diet and increasing your physical activity will lead to overall improvements in health that will benefit you on many different levels. Weight loss achieved through improved diet and exercise, for example, can help control your blood pressure and blood sugar levels without the need for additional medications and their possible accompanying side effects.

There are currently six classes of drugs used to modify lipid levels (see table 2.4). They each have varying effects: some are primarily used to lower LDL-C, while others predominantly alter levels of triglycerides and HDL-C. Each may be prescribed individually or in combination with another class of drug.

Table 2.4. Effects of Drug Classes on Lipids[20]

Drug Class	Total C	LDL-C	HDL-C	Triglycerides
Statins	↓ 15% – 60%	↓ 21% – 63%	↑ 5% – 15%	↓ 10% – 37%
Bile acid resins	↓ 20%	↓ 15% – 25%	↑ 3% – 5%	Variable
Cholesterol absorption inhibitors	↓ 13%	↓ 19%	↑ 3%	↓ 8%
Nicotinic acid	↓ 25%	↓ 5% – 25%	↑ 15% – 35%	↓ 20% – 50%
Fibric acid derivatives	↓ 15%	Variable	↑ 10% – 20%	↓ 20% – 50%
Omega-3 fatty acids	N/A	N/A	N/A	↓ 35% – 50%

Statins

Statins are the most popular and effective lipid-lowering drug currently available. They are technically called *HMG-CoA reductase inhibitors*. They act by interfering with the body's ability to manufacture its own cholesterol in the liver. As cholesterol levels in the liver drop, LDL-C is drawn out of the blood through special receptors in the liver called LDL receptors. This results in decreased cholesterol levels in the blood.

Statins are primarily used to lower LDL-C (21–63 percent decrease). They can also reduce triglycerides (10–37 percent decrease) and modestly increase HDL-C levels (5–15 percent increase). There are a variety of statins available in the United States: atorvastatin (Lipitor®), fluvastatin (Lescol®), lovastatin (Mevacor®, Altoprev®), pitavastatin (Livalo®), pravastatin (Pravachol®), rosuvastatin (Crestor®), and simvastatin (Zocor®). Many are now available in generic form.

The statins all work in the same way and have similar effects on lipid levels. However, there are differences in how each drug is used and in their strength. Your doctor will decide which statin is the most appropriate for you. In general, statins are easy to take, and they have minimal side effects and excellent safety records. Studies have shown that for every 39 mg/dL reduction in LDL-C obtained with a statin drug, the risk of dying from heart disease, having a heart attack or stroke, or undergoing a hospital procedure to clear blocked arteries within a five-year period decreases by about 20 percent.[21] Statins protect against heart disease regardless of what your initial LDL-C level is, so if you start out with an LDL-C of 190 mg/dL and reduce it by 39 mg/dL, you will experience the same proportional reduction in risk as someone with an initial LDL-C of 100 mg/dL.

Rare side effects with statins have included muscle ailments, so alert your physician if you experience any unexplained muscle weakness or pain. Measures of *creatine kinase* (CK), an enzyme that indicates muscle damage, are used to diagnose statin-related muscle disease. *Myopathy* is muscle pain, soreness, or weakness accompanied by creatine kinase levels exceeding ten times the upper limit of normal; it occurs in approximately 1 in 10,000 patients treated with statins.[22] Very rarely, myopathy can progress to *rhabdomyolysis*, which is the rapid breakdown of skeletal muscle accompanied by creatine kinase levels exceeding forty times the upper limit of normal. Typically, any muscular symptoms that arise disappear after stopping the statin. The risk for muscular side effects is increased by high statin doses and by interactions with certain other drugs, so make sure to tell your physician what other medications you are currently taking. A recent study called SEARCH found that simvastatin at the highest dose (80 mg/day) increased risk for myopathy, so the Food and Drug Administration (FDA) recommends that no new patients be prescribed simvastatin at this dose.[23]

Statins are not generally recommended in patients with confirmed or suspected liver disease since they can occasionally affect liver function. Before taking a statin, your physician will order routine blood tests to measure your liver enzymes, and these levels will be monitored periodically. Statins are also not used in women who are pregnant, likely to become pregnant, or breast-feeding, since cholesterol is essential to fetal development and statins are excreted in breast milk.

A recent discovery is that statins may increase the risk of a person developing diabetes by about 9 percent.[24] This means that one person may develop diabetes as a side effect of a statin for every 255 people treated with the drug for four years, while 5.4 heart attacks or deaths from coronary causes may be prevented. The risk for developing diabetes is relatively low, considering how effective statins are at reducing cardiovascular risk. People who are prescribed statins are considered to be at high to moderate risk for developing heart disease, so the cardiovascular benefits of statins outweigh the risk of developing diabetes in these individuals.

Bile Acid Resins

Bile acid resins, also called resins or bile acid sequestrants, are primarily used for LDL-C reduction (15–25 percent decrease). They may slightly increase HDL-C (3–5 percent increase) and have variable effects on triglyceride levels. They work by binding to bile acids in the intestines, which increases bile acid excretion from the body. As levels of bile acid drop, the liver converts more cholesterol to bile acids, resulting in less cholesterol in the liver. Decreased cholesterol levels in the liver lead to more LDL-C being drawn out of the blood through the liver's LDL receptors. The overall result is a decrease in cholesterol levels in the blood.

There are three kinds of resins: cholestyramine (LoCholest®, Questran®, Prevalite®), colestipol (Cholestid®), and colesevelam (WelChol®). Colesevelam is the newest resin and was specially designed to reduce the gastrointestinal side effects common to this class of drug. In 2008 colesevelam was also approved for glucose (blood sugar) control in patients with diabetes.

The resins do not seem to enter the bloodstream. However, constipation, bloating, gas, and heartburn are common side effects. Increasing consumption of fluids and fiber can help relieve constipation, as can stool softeners. "Light" (containing artificial sweetener instead of sugar) and tablet preparations are also available. Side effects, if they occur, usually lessen over time. Resins can interfere with the absorption of other medications in the intestine. Make sure to discuss with your physician when to take other medications if you are prescribed a resin.

Cholesterol Absorption Inhibitors

Cholesterol absorption inhibitors are the newest class of lipid-lowering drug. Only one agent in this class, ezetimibe (Zetia®), has been approved. There is also a combination agent incorporating ezetimibe and simvastatin (Vytorin®). Ezetimibe works by decreasing the absorption of dietary cholesterol from the intestines. This results in decreased cholesterol levels in the liver and a subsequent removal of cholesterol from the blood. Ezetimibe alone reduces LDL-C by approximately 19 percent, and it has modest effects on HDL-C (3 percent increase) and triglycerides (8 percent decrease). When it is combined with a statin, the effect of both drugs appears additive, and LDL-C levels can be reduced by as much as 60 percent. Ezetimibe is generally used in people who have trouble reaching their LDL-C target with one drug alone or who do not tolerate statins.

Since ezetimibe is a newer drug and was introduced in the United States in 2006, there is little hard evidence yet that it reduces clinical outcomes such as heart attack and stroke. During 2008–2009, ezetimibe received a lot of attention in the press due to the results of three trials—ENHANCE, SEAS, and ARBITER 6-HALTS—that raised questions about ezetimibe's ability to reduce cardiovascular risk as much as established drugs, such as statins and nicotinic acid.[25] The question remains unresolved, and a large ongoing study with ezetimibe in patients with heart disease should provide more data in a few years. One recent trial did find that the combination of ezetimibe and a statin reduced cardiovascular events in patients with advanced chronic kidney disease, a population that previously had not been shown to benefit significantly from cholesterol-lowering treatment.[26] Until more information is known, ezetimibe has been shown to reduce LDL-C levels substantially and is considered a safe alternative for patients who do not tolerate statins or who need further reductions in LDL-C after starting statin therapy.

Nicotinic Acid

Nicotinic acid, or niacin, is a B vitamin that, at high doses, is effective at lowering LDL-C (5–25 percent decrease) and triglycerides (20–50 percent decrease) and at raising HDL-C (15–35 percent increase) levels. It can also reduce levels of Lp(a) by about 25 percent. Its primary effect is to decrease the production of VLDL (the primary carrier of triglycerides) by the liver, which subsequently affects the levels of other lipoproteins. It also decreases the breakdown of triglycerides to fatty acids within the body's fat reserves. As a result, fewer fatty acids are transported back to the liver. Fatty acids are needed to synthesize VLDL in the liver, so the levels of other lipoproteins are further altered.

Nicotinic acid at low doses can be purchased over the counter, although you should not take nicotinic acid supplements for cholesterol reduction without a doctor's supervision. Nicotinic acid is also available in a prescription extended-release formulation (Niaspan®), which may reduce some of the side effects associated with this class of drug. In addition, there are two combination drugs that combine extended-release nicotinic acid with a statin: niacin/lovastatin (Advicor®) and niacin/simvastatin (Simcor®). Nicotinic acid is not the same as nicotinamide, which is sometimes called niacin but does not lower cholesterol.

Many patients experience uncomfortable side effects with the use of nicotinic acid. These side effects commonly include flushing (turning red) and tingling sensations in the face, as well as itching and dry skin. Starting at a low dosage of nicotinic acid and gradually increasing it tends to lessen these side effects. Taking aspirin or other over-the-counter, anti-inflammatory pain medications can also reduce flushing. In Europe, a drug called laropiprant, which is not currently approved in the United States, can be combined with nicotinic acid to decrease the flushing response. It works by interfering with *prostaglandin*, a compound that is activated by nicotinic acid and that causes blood vessels to dilate, leading to flushing. Other less common side effects of nicotinic acid include nausea, vomiting, diarrhea, alterations in liver function, and darkening of the skin in body folds and creases, especially in the armpits (a condition called *acanthosis nigricans*). Side effects usually disappear after discontinuing nicotinic acid.

Nicotinic acid can worsen glucose intolerance (difficulty regulating blood sugar levels) and should be used with caution in people with diabetes. Individuals with liver disease, peptic ulcers, or a history of gout should also be carefully monitored.

Fibrates

Fibrates, or fibric acid derivatives, are usually well tolerated and are effective in lowering triglycerides (20–50 percent decrease) and raising HDL-C levels (10–20 percent increase). Their effect on LDL-C levels is variable: they can substantially lower them, but in some cases they may even raise them, depending on the level of triglycerides. They work by activating many different molecular pathways that affect levels of triglycerides and HDL-C. One of their effects is to increase the breakdown of triglyceride-rich lipoproteins. They also increase the particle size of small dense LDL. The fibrates available in the United States are gemfibrozil (Lopid®) and fenofibrate (Lipofen®, Lofibra®, Tricor®, Trilipix®).

Gastrointestinal side effects may occur in up to 5 percent of people taking fibrates. In rare cases, they may affect liver function. Fibrates are not used in patients with liver or severe kidney disease, or in patients with gallbladder disease. They can interfere with oral anticoagulants (anticlotting drugs), so people taking warfarin may need to have their dosages reduced. Muscle ailments are rare when fibrates are taken as the only lipid-lowering drug, but when they are taken in combination with a statin, the risk for muscular side effects increases. Notify your doctor if you are prescribed a statin/fibrate combination and muscular pain or weakness occur.

Omega-3 Fatty Acids

Omega-3 fatty acids are found in fish oil and have been shown to reduce cardiovascular risk when consumed both as fish and as a dietary supplement. In addition to being part of an overall healthy diet (see the section in this chapter on diet), omega-3 fatty acids are available in a prescription-strength formulation for the treatment of high triglycerides (Lovaza®). This formulation contains a combination of eicosapentaenoic acid (EPA) and docosahexaenoic acid (DHA), which are the omega-3 fatty acids believed to be particularly beneficial to the heart. At a dose of 4 grams per day, which is much higher than can be obtained simply by eating fish, prescription-strength omega-3 fatty acids can reduce triglycerides by 35 to 50 percent in patients with very high triglyceride levels ($\geq$ 500 mg/dL). In some cases, they can increase LDL-C levels, so these levels need to be monitored. Common side effects include gastrointestinal complaints, such as moderate diarrhea. Before taking fish oil supplements to reduce cardiovascular risk or triglycerides, first consult a physician.

Blood Pressure

The dramatic phrase "the silent killer" is used frequently to describe high blood pressure, or hypertension. Hypertension earned this nickname by having no noticeable symptoms: a person can have high blood pressure for years without knowing it. If hypertension is ignored and goes undiagnosed and untreated, it can have serious, even deadly, consequences (see figure 2.1). It is a major risk factor for cerebrovascular disease (stroke and brain aneurysms), and it significantly increases the risk for kidney failure and coronary artery disease. Uncontrolled hypertension causes the heart to increase the energy required for pumping, and the heart may enlarge to meet that demand. Hypertension increases aneurysm formation and can cause large arteries to rupture. The arteries and smaller arterioles may lose their elasticity and harden from the scarring caused by increased pressure against their inner walls, gradually becoming less able to supply the tissues they serve with needed blood. The longer blood pressure remains high, the greater the risk for damage to body organs such as the kidney. Hardened and narrowed arteries can also lead to the formation of blood clots, which can cause heart attacks and strokes. Severely high blood pressure may cause headaches and bleeding into the blood vessels of the eye, resulting in damage to the retina or loss of eyesight.

According to the American Heart Association, hypertension currently affects approximately one in three adults in the United States.[27] Blood pressure guidelines for adults classify blood pressure in stages: normal, prehypertension, stage 1 hypertension, and stage 2 hypertension (see table 2.5). High blood pressure is considered to be present when *systolic blood pressure* (the first number in a reading) is greater than 140 mm Hg or *diastolic blood pressure* (the second number in a reading) is greater than 90 mm Hg, based on the average of two or more readings. Blood pressure can vary widely and is affected by a variety of factors, such as the stress of being at the doctor's office, excitement, recent exercise, or some illnesses and medications, so accurate diagnosis of hypertension requires at least two visits to the doctor after an initial screening.

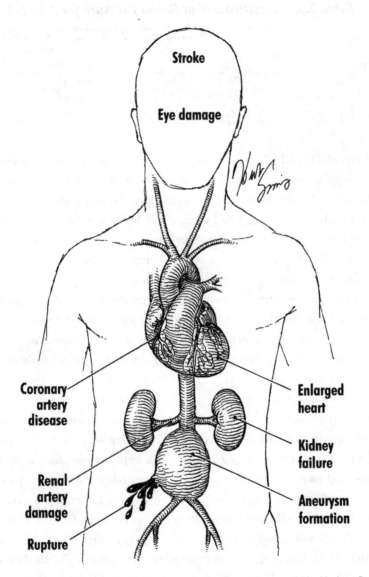

Figure 2.1. Potential consequences of hypertension. *Illustration created by Herbert R. Smith Jr.*

Table 2.5.   Classification of Blood Pressure for Adults[28]

BP Classification	Systolic Blood Pressure (mm Hg)	Diastolic Blood Pressure (mm Hg)
Normal	< 120	And < 80
Prehypertension	120–139	Or 80–89
Stage 1 hypertension	140–159	Or 90–99
Stage 2 hypertension	≥ 160	Or ≥ 100

Between 90 and 95 percent of people with hypertension have essential (or primary) hypertension, which means that it is not associated with any known cause. Primary hypertension cannot often be cured, but it can be controlled with lifestyle changes and medication. Secondary hypertension results from the presence of a specific disease or medical condition (including kidney disease, primary hyperaldosteronism, renal artery stenosis, coarctation of the aorta, Cushing's disease, hyperthyroidism, or pregnancy). Once the underlying disease or condition is identified and resolved, secondary high blood pressure will usually disappear. Low blood pressure, or *hypotension*, can be a chronic condition and is generally not a serious health problem. An exception is severe postural hypotension, in which blood pressure drops suddenly when an individual moves from a sitting or lying position to a standing one, causing lightheadedness or fainting.

While the exact causes of many cases of hypertension cannot be identified, there are specific, often interrelated risk factors that seem to play important roles in its development. Some risk factors for hypertension, such as heredity, age, sex, and race, cannot be controlled. An individual who has a parent or other close relative with hypertension is more likely to develop it eventually than an individual with no family history of hypertension. Blood pressure risk changes by age and occurs more commonly after age thirty. From young adulthood to early middle age, men are more likely to develop high blood pressure; from middle age to old age, hypertension is more likely to affect women. Women who take oral contraceptives are two to three times more likely to develop high blood pressure, especially if they are obese, smoke, or are older in age, compared to women not taking them.

Hypertension can sometimes develop in women with otherwise normal blood pressure during the last three months of pregnancy. If left untreated, this condition can be dangerous to both the mother and the baby. Hypertension that develops during pregnancy usually disappears after delivery. If it does not, it should be medically treated and controlled in the same way as other types of hypertension. A woman who already has hypertension when she becomes pregnant should be carefully monitored by a physician. Pregnancy may or may not make hypertension more severe, but with careful treatment, a woman should be able to have a normal pregnancy and a normal baby.

The risk for high blood pressure is strongly affected by race. African Americans have some of the highest rates of high blood pressure in the world. During 2005 through 2008, approximately 43 percent of African Americans had high blood pressure, compared to 30 percent of whites.[29] In addition, African Americans develop high blood pressure at an earlier age than whites, and their blood pressure elevations are more severe. They have a 1.8 times greater rate of fatal stroke, a 1.3 times greater rate of nonfatal stroke, and a 1.5 times greater rate of heart disease deaths, due in large part to higher rates of high blood pressure.[30]

Lifestyle Changes

High blood pressure can often be prevented through exercise and the control of weight, sodium intake, and alcohol consumption. The risk factors for hypertension that can be modified (obesity, sedentary lifestyle, high sodium, and alcohol intake) are also the areas that a doctor will ask you to focus on should you develop hypertension. Most cases of high blood pressure cannot be cured; however, the good news is that it can be controlled by lifestyle changes and, when necessary, medication. Unless there is an immediate need for medication because of severe hypertension or other medical complications, most patients will be advised to try to lower their blood pressure levels by making lifestyle changes first. For many otherwise healthy individuals with stage 1 hypertension, lifestyle modifications may lower their blood pressure to a normal level.

The following section describes risk factors for hypertension related to lifestyle, and it suggests changes that can help to lower your blood pressure or prevent high blood pressure in the first place (also see the sections in this chapter on obesity, physical inactivity, and diet).

Obesity

Obesity is closely linked with hypertension because it causes the heart to struggle to supply excess tissue with blood. Controlling weight is an important factor in preventing and treating high blood pressure, and blood pressure has been found to decrease in proportion to weight loss. Weight loss has also been found to improve the effectiveness of blood pressure medications.

> *Goal.* Reach and maintain a desirable body weight. Your body mass index (BMI) should be between 18.5 and 24.9 kg/m². Go to the National Institutes of Health website (http://www.nhlbisupport.com/bmi/) to calculate your BMI by entering your height and weight using either standard or metric measures. Weight loss of about ten pounds can be expected to lower systolic blood pressure by around 3–8 mm Hg.

Sedentary Lifestyle

Being sedentary—inactive—can be dangerous to your health. People who are sedentary are more likely to develop hypertension than those who are active. Those who become active typically experience a modest decrease in their blood pressure, whether or not they lose weight. Low- to moderate-intensity exercise is as effective as high-intensity exercise in reducing blood pressure.

> *Goal.* Exercise regularly. Taking part in aerobic physical activity every day is more likely to lower blood pressure than exercising only a few times per week. Brisk walking for at least thirty minutes per day on most days of the week is a good starting point and can be expected to reduce systolic blood pressure by as much as 10 mm Hg. Before beginning an exercise program, be sure to check with your physician.

Alcohol Consumption

Excessive alcohol consumption can raise blood pressure and can cause resistance to high blood pressure medications. Alcohol intake of three or more drinks at a time temporarily increases blood pressure, and repeated heavy drinking can elevate blood pressure long-term. Reducing alcohol consumption has been found to lower blood pressure in people with normal and high blood pressure levels, as well as in alcoholics and nonalcoholics. For those who drink, lowering alcohol intake may also help prevent the development of high blood pressure in the first place. People with hypertension who choose to drink alcoholic beverages should do so only in moderation.

> *Goal.* Limit alcohol intake to no more than two drinks per day for most men and to no more than one drink per day for women and lighter-weight persons. One drink is equal to 0.5 ounces or 15 milliliter of ethanol (12 ounces of beer, 5 ounces of wine, or 1.5 ounces of eighty-proof whiskey). Switching to moderate alcohol consumption can reduce systolic blood pressure by 2–4 mm Hg.

Sodium Intake

A strong link connects sodium consumption to blood pressure. Sodium causes the body to retain extra fluid, which puts a greater burden on the heart and narrows blood vessels; this, in turn, raises blood pressure. A diet that is high in sodium also decreases the effectiveness of medications used to treat high blood pressure. Sodium is obtained primarily from sodium chloride, or common table salt, although it is also found in large amounts in baking powder, monosodium glutamate (MSG), and soy sauce. About 75 percent of the sodium in the American diet can be attributed to the salt and other sodium compounds added to food during processing.

> *Goal.* For people without hypertension, reduce sodium intake to 2,300 milligrams or less per day (the equivalent of

about one teaspoon of table salt). For people with hypertension, diabetes, or chronic kidney disease, or who are African American or over the age of fifty, aim for a daily sodium intake of 1,500 milligrams or less (slightly less than two-thirds of a teaspoon of table salt). According to the CDC, nine out of ten US adults consume too much sodium, with an average daily sodium intake of approximately 3,500 milligrams.[31] Reducing sodium intake can be expected to lower systolic blood pressure by 2–8 mm Hg.

Overall Healthy Diet

The DASH (Dietary Approaches to Stop Hypertension) diet is recommended to many people with hypertension or prehypertension (see the section in this chapter on diet), and it is endorsed by many national health organizations, including the American Heart Association and the National Institutes for Health (http://www.nhlbi.nih.gov/health/public/heart/hbp/dash/). It is a low-sodium diet rich in fruits and vegetables that incorporates low-fat or nonfat dairy products. Many fruits and vegetables are high in potassium, which can protect against the development of high blood pressure and help keep levels as low as possible. Foods high in potassium and low in sodium include bananas, potatoes, beans, cantaloupes, and yogurt.

> *Goal.* Consume an overall healthy diet rich in fruits and vegetables and low in fat and sodium. The DASH diet is especially recommended for people trying to control their high blood pressure. Numerous recipes that follow the DASH diet are available online and in bookstores.

Antihypertensive Medications

If lifestyle changes are not effective in lowering blood pressure, physicians may then prescribe medication to control high blood pressure. Lifestyle modifications should be ongoing, as they can cause antihypertensive medications to work more effectively. In clinical trials, antihypertensive medications have been shown to reduce the risk of heart attack by 20 to 25 percent, of stroke by 35 to 40 percent, and of heart failure by more than 50 percent.[32] For individuals with stage 1 hypertension and additional cardiovascular risk factors, reducing systolic blood pressure by 12 mm Hg over ten years is estimated to prevent one death for every eleven people treated with blood pressure-lowering medication.

Blood pressure control can be achieved with several different types of medication. A physician frequently will prescribe more than one type of antihypertensive medication for maximal control. Diuretics, for example, enhance the effect of other antihypertensive medications when used in combination. Patients may react differently to each of these medications, and some may experience side effects. Determining the medication or combination of medications that will most effectively lower your blood pressure with the fewest side effects may take time. Side effects can often be moderated or eliminated by lowering dosage or by substituting another medication. After beginning a new antihypertensive medication, be sure to report any new or unusual symptoms to your physician.

Thiazide diuretics are generally the first choice of therapy, either alone or in combination, unless you have a history of heart failure, heart attack, diabetes, chronic kidney disease, stroke, or high cardiovascular risk. If you have one of these conditions, a physician may prescribe one of the other classes of drug for initial therapy.

Diuretics

Diuretics are often the first type of medication prescribed for treatment of hypertension. Diuretics act on the kidneys, helping to remove excess water and salt from the body. Diuretics pull water from tissues, relieving fluid buildup (edema), and help convert the water to urine. This fluid removal reduces blood volume. Lower circulating blood volume allows blood pressure to drop, and less strain is put on the heart.

In several clinical trials, diuretics have been shown to reduce stroke, heart disease, and death compared to placebo, particularly in elderly and black patients.[33] Diuretics are inexpensive and are especially effective in combination with other antihypertensive drugs, including beta-blockers, angiotensin-converting enzyme (ACE) inhibitors, and angiotensin receptor blockers (ARBs). At high doses, diuretics can adversely affect the lipid profile and may increase the risk of developing diabetes. They have the potential to cause low blood pressure, or hypotension, which is a particular concern for older people as it can lead to dizziness or a feeling of faintness, thereby increasing the risk for falls. Diuretics can cause a decrease in potassium levels and can cause impotence in men, which is a relatively common side effect.

Several types of diuretics are available. These include thiazide, loop, and potassium-sparing agents. Side effects vary by class of drug. Thiazide diuretics are the most common and the type generally recommended as initial therapy for most patients. However, they remove potassium along with other minerals. Excessive potassium loss can cause muscle cramps, weakness, and impotence, and it may trigger irregular heartbeats. Your doctor may advise you to take potassium supplements or to consume high-potassium foods, such as bananas and fruit juices. Alternatively, a potassium-sparing diuretic, ACE inhibitor, or ARB can be prescribed along with the thiazide diuretic to prevent potassium loss. At high doses, thiazide medications can increase LDL-C and triglyceride levels, and they have also been associated with elevations in blood sugar and uric acid in susceptible individuals, including some diabetics and people at risk for developing gout.

Loop diuretics are fast-acting agents that promote a high urine output over several hours. Like thiazide preparations, loop diuretics remove potassium. They can also deplete other *electrolytes* (minerals that help regulate fluid balance) and, in fact, are used to reduce high blood calcium levels (whereas thiazides can raise blood calcium). In high dosages, loop diuretics may affect hearing and can increase LDL-C.

Unlike thiazide diuretics, potassium-sparing diuretics, as the name suggests, preserve potassium, and they do not significantly alter lipid levels. Potassium-sparing agents typically are given in combination with another type of diuretic. Aldosterone antagonists are a type of potassium-sparing agent that is used to treat hypertensive patients with heart failure or following a heart attack. They may also be useful in patients with hypertension who do not respond well to other drug treatment.

Beta-Blockers

If diuretics are not effective in lowering blood pressure, a beta-adrenergic blocker, called beta-blocker for short, may be considered as a second choice, either alone or in combination. Beta-blockers work by decreasing the heart rate and the force of the heart's contractions. They also affect *renin* (an enzyme in the kidney that helps regulate fluid balance and blood vessel contraction), and they trigger the release of prostaglandins (substances that help to relax and widen blood vessels). Side effects that have been linked with beta-blockers include fatigue and shortness of breath at low levels of exertion, increases in body weight, and reduced awareness of symptoms of hypoglycemia (low blood sugar) in individuals with diabetes. Beta-blockers may also increase triglycerides and lower levels of HDL-C.

Calcium Channel Blockers

Calcium channel blockers (CCBs) lower blood pressure by relaxing and widening blood vessels, and they decrease the resistance from blood flow throughout the body's vessels. They are equal to the other drug classes in reducing blood pressure, but they are better in protecting against stroke. CCBs are especially effective in elderly and African American patients. They act independently of salt intake. For individuals with hypertension and high cholesterol, there is a combination drug available that incorporates the CCB amlodipine with the statin drug atorvastatin (Caduet®). The ASCOT-LLA trial showed that this combination reduced cardiovascular events in hypertensive patients at high risk for developing heart disease.[34]

CCBs are more expensive than diuretics, but unlike diuretics, they do not significantly affect blood sugar, electrolytes, or blood lipid levels. Individuals who are determined to be at high risk for cardiovascular disease or who have diabetes are generally prescribed CCBs. However, CCBs may increase the risk of heart failure in some patients. Other side effects are associated with low blood pressure, such as headaches and dizziness, and may also include swelling of the ankles (edema).

ACE Inhibitors

Angiotensin-converting enzyme (ACE) is present in blood vessel walls and in the blood. Under normal circumstances, ACE converts a chemical called angiotensin I to *angiotensin II*, a substance that induces blood vessels to constrict. By blocking ACE, ACE inhibitors shut down production of angiotensin II, allowing blood vessels to relax and dilate.

ACE inhibitors can dramatically reduce blood pressure in cases of malignant hypertension (when blood pressure rises suddenly to extremely high levels, which can cause organ damage if left untreated). It is also effective in people with less extreme blood pressure elevations. When used by itself for treatment of hypertension, it is important to restrict salt intake to maximize the drug's effectiveness. In general, African American patients, particularly those who are elderly, do not respond as well to ACE inhibitors as white patients; African Americans may be given higher doses or an ACE inhibitor in combination with a thiazide diuretic. ACE inhibitors do not alter glucose (blood sugar) or cholesterol levels and, in fact, may lessen the development of diabetes in hypertensive patients.

One of the most common side effects associated with ACE inhibitors is a dry cough, which may occur in about 10 percent of patients. The cough is believed to be caused by increased levels of bradykinin and prostaglandins, which help to relax and dilate blood vessels. Switching to another class of drug, such as an ARB, can lessen the cough. In addition, ACE inhibitors can cause hypotension or low blood pressure, can elevate potassium levels, and have been known to worsen certain kidney conditions. ACE inhibitors should not be used during pregnancy.

Angiotensin Receptor Blockers

ARBs are a newer drug class that acts on the receptor for angiotensin II. These drugs do not block ACE, do not increase bradykinin levels, and generally are not associated with a cough. They are the fastest growing class of antihypertensive drug in the United States and in Europe, but they are also generally more expensive. ARBs should not be used during pregnancy. People with heart failure, diabetes, and chronic kidney disease are often prescribed this class of drug. ARBs are associated with few side effects.

Direct Renin Inhibitors

Direct renin inhibitors are the most recently approved class of antihypertensive medication. They work by blocking renin, an enzyme in the kidney, which then causes blood vessels to relax and widen. There is currently only one drug in this class available in the United States, called aliskiren (Tekturna®). It can be used in combination with other blood pressure medications. The most common side effect is diarrhea; rare side effects include a rash or swelling in the face, throat, or limbs. Direct renin inhibitors should not be used during pregnancy.

Cigarette Smoking

Cigarette smokers are two to three times more likely to die of heart disease than nonsmokers. Currently, approximately 443,000 people in the United States die from smoking-related diseases each year, and 30 percent of these deaths are related to cardiovascular disease.[35] Cigarette smoking also doubles the risk for stroke. Female smokers are ten times more likely to develop peripheral artery disease in which vessels carrying blood to the arms and legs narrow and fail to deliver needed oxygen and nutrients. Women who smoke while taking oral contraceptives are at even greater risk for developing cardiovascular disease. On average, smokers die fourteen years earlier than nonsmokers.

In addition to its damaging effects on the lungs, smoking harms the cardiovascular system by making the blood more likely to clot. It increases the amount of carbon monoxide in the blood, which reduces the amount of oxygen that can reach the body's cells. Smoking also increases blood pressure and decreases HDL-C levels. The more cigarettes you smoke, the more that your risk for developing cardiovascular disease is increased.

Secondhand smoke increases the risk of dying from premature heart disease, and it increases the risk for developing CHD by 25 to 30 percent.[36] Approximately 126 million nonsmoking people are exposed to secondhand smoke, including 60 percent of all children, who may be exposed to it both at home and at other locations. If you already have heart disease, exposure to secondhand smoke can make a heart attack more severe than it would have been otherwise.

More than four in five smokers in the United States say they want to quit. If you are a smoker, it may help you quit if you know that your increased risk for heart disease is reduced by half within one year after quitting (see table 2.6). Studies have shown that this appears to hold true regardless of how long you smoked or how many cigarettes you smoked daily. Men who quit smoking between the ages of thirty-five and thirty-nine years add an average of five years to their life, while women in this age group who quit add three years. Patients who are encouraged by a doctor to quit are more likely to be successful at quitting. So if your doctor hasn't told you to quit, please take our advice to stop now.

Whether you stop "cold turkey" (withdrawing from smoking all at once), gradually, or with nicotine replacement therapy or prescription medication, the important issue is deciding to quit. Be aware that stopping smoking can lead to nicotine withdrawal symptoms, which may begin within a few hours of the last cigarette. Withdrawal symptoms are strongest about two to three days after quitting, when most of the nicotine has left the body, but they generally disappear after a few days or up to several weeks. According to the American Cancer Society, withdrawal symptoms can include any of the following:

- Dizziness
- Depression or anxiety
- Irritability or feelings of frustration, impatience, and anger
- Sleep disturbances
- Restlessness or trouble concentrating
- Headaches
- Tiredness
- Increased appetite and weight gain

Stopping smoking can cause physical withdrawal symptoms, but it can also be difficult psychologically. For these reasons, it is important to use all the resources available to help you quit.

Table 2.6. When Smokers Quit—Benefits of Quitting Over Time

20 minutes after quitting: Your heart rate and blood pressure drops.
(Effect of Smoking on Arterial Stiffness and Pulse Pressure Amplification,
Mahmud, A, Feely, J. 2003. *Hypertension*:41:183.)

12 hours after quitting: The carbon monoxide level in your blood drops to normal.
(*US Surgeon General's Report*, 1988, p. 202)

2 weeks to 3 months after quitting: Your circulation improves, and your lung
function increases.
(*US Surgeon General's Report*, 1990, pp. 193, 194,196, 285, 323)

1 to 9 months after quitting: Coughing and shortness of breath decrease;
cilia (tiny hair-like structures that move mucus out of the lungs) regain normal
function in the lungs, increasing the ability to handle mucus, clean the lungs, and
reduce the risk of infection.
(*US Surgeon General's Report*, 1990, pp. 285-287, 304)

1 year after quitting: The excess risk of coronary heart disease is half that of a
smoker's.
(*US Surgeon General's Report*, 1990, p. vi)

5 years after quitting: Your stroke risk is reduced to that of a nonsmoker 5 to 15
years after quitting.
(*US Surgeon General's Report*, 1990, p. vi)

10 years after quitting: The lung cancer death rate is about half that of a
continuing smoker's. The risk of cancer of the mouth, throat, esophagus, bladder,
cervix, and pancreas decreases.
(*US Surgeon General's Report*, 1990, pp. vi, 131, 148, 152, 155, 164, 166)

15 years after quitting: The risk of coronary heart disease is that of a
non-smoker's.
(*US Surgeon General's Report*, 1990, p. vi)

How to Quit Smoking

Beginning in 2008, all states have a free telephone counseling program to help smokers quit. For example, the American Cancer Society has a program called Quitline that links callers with trained counselors in your area. You can call 1-800-QUIT-NOW from anywhere to receive information in your state. Counselors may suggest a combination of medication, local classes, self-help brochures, and a support network. People who use telephone counseling are twice as likely to quit smoking as those who don't.

Nicotine replacement therapy is available with and without a prescription and can be helpful in reducing withdrawal symptoms. The best time to start nicotine replacement therapy is when you first quit. You do not need to wait any specific length of time after your last cigarette, although you should generally not smoke while wearing a nicotine patch. National guidelines recommend the use of nicotine replacement therapy for all adult smokers, although pregnant women and people with cardiovascular disease should only begin these medications under a physician's supervision. People who smoke fewer than ten cigarettes per day should also consult a physician, as nicotine replacement therapy has not been shown to help light smokers to quit. Combining nicotine replacement therapy with a stop-smoking program has been shown to double the chances of quitting smoking permanently.

There are currently five types of approved nicotine replacement therapy.

Nicotine Patches

Nicotine patches, also referred to as transdermal nicotine systems, evenly administer a continuous dose of nicotine over either a sixteen-hour or twenty-four-hour period. There are over-the-counter and prescription varieties. The sixteen-hour patch is good for light-to-average smokers and may cause fewer side effects. The twenty-four-hour patch helps with early-morning withdrawal but may have increased side effects. Depending on body size, a full-strength patch (15–22 mg) should be used for four weeks before switching to a weaker patch (5–14 mg) for four weeks. It is recommended that the patch be used for a total of three to five months.

Some potential side effects of the nicotine patch include skin irritation, dizziness, racing heartbeat, sleep problems, headache, nausea, vomiting, or muscle aches and stiffness. If you have side effects, consider switching to a different brand or a weaker patch.

Nicotine Gum

With this method, nicotine is absorbed through the mucus membranes in the mouth. Carrying nicotine gum is easy and leaves control of the dosage in the hands of the person trying to quit. People who need something to chew or to occupy their hands, who want to control cravings when they occur, or who smoke at irregular intervals may find nicotine gum their best choice. People with sensitive skin may also prefer gum to the patch. Nicotine gum is available without a prescription and comes in 2-milligram and 4-milligram strengths. It is generally sugar-free. Do not chew more than twenty pieces of gum in one day. Nicotine gum is generally recommended for one to three months, up to a maximum of six months.

Possible side effects of nicotine gum include a bad taste, throat irritation, mouth sores, hiccups, nausea, jaw discomfort, or a racing heartbeat. Some of these symptoms may result from swallowing the nicotine or chewing too fast. A possible disadvantage of nicotine gum is long-term dependence, although chewing the gum is probably less dangerous than starting to smoke again.

Nicotine Nasal Spray

When one uses the nasal spray, nicotine is absorbed through the nose and delivered to the bloodstream. It is available only by prescription. Like the gum, the nasal spray lets you control cravings when they occur. However, there is also the risk of long-term dependence. It is recommended that the nasal spray be prescribed for three months at a time, up to a maximum of six months. Possible side effects include nasal irritation, runny nose, watery eyes, sneezing, throat irritation, and coughing. People with asthma, allergies, nasal polyps, or sinus problems may want to consider another form of nicotine replacement therapy in consultation with their physician.

Nicotine Inhalers

Nicotine inhalers are the method of quitting smoking that is most like smoking a cigarette. The inhaler is a thin, plastic tube with a nicotine cartridge inside that emits a nicotine vapor. Most of the nicotine vapor is delivered to the mouth, unlike other inhalers that mostly deliver medicine to the lungs. Nicotine inhalers are only available by prescription and are currently the most expensive form of nicotine replacement therapy. The recommended dose is between six and sixteen cartridges per day for up to six months. Common side effects such as coughing, throat irritation, and upset stomach may occur when you first begin using the inhaler.

Nicotine Lozenges

Nicotine lozenges are available over the counter and are the newest form of nicotine replacement therapy. They are available in 2-milligram and 4-milligram strengths, and it is recommended that they be used as part of a twelve-week smoking cessation program. You should not use more than twenty lozenges per day, and the lozenges should be allowed to dissolve fully in the mouth. Possible side effects include trouble sleeping, nausea, hiccups, coughing, heartburn, headache, and gas. They are generally sugar-free.

***

There are also prescription medications that do not contain nicotine that can help people stop smoking. Bupropion (Zyban®) is an extended-release antidepressant that reduces symptoms of nicotine withdrawal by acting on chemicals in the brain related to nicotine craving. It can be used alone or in combination with nicotine replacement therapy. Varenicline (Chantix®) is a newer prescription medication that interferes with nicotine receptors in the brain. It works by lessening the pleasurable physical effects produced by smoking, and it reduces the symptoms of nicotine withdrawal. Varenicline has been shown to double the chances of quitting. Since it is a newer drug, it is not yet clear whether it is safe to use varenicline in combination with nicotine replacement therapy. In the past few years, both bupropion and varenicline have been associated with reports of suicide in patients trying to stop smoking, and the FDA has issued a warning that people taking these drugs should be watched closely for signs of serious mental illness.[37] Studies investigating the potential mental health risks of bupropion and varenicline are ongoing.

Many people worry about weight gain with smoking cessation. Some smokers may gain some weight, in part because their senses of taste and smell are improved and they enjoy food more. But the average weight gain is usually less than ten pounds. You can avoid weight gain by eating a healthy, low-fat diet and using carrot sticks, raisins, or apples for oral substitutes. Regular physical activity, such as walking, will help you keep busy, relax, and improve your overall fitness.

Do whatever works for you to quit smoking, and don't feel alone when you are discouraged. Only about 4 to 7 percent of people can quit smoking by themselves, without medication or other support.[38] About 25 to 33 percent of smokers who use medicines to help them quit smoking remain smoke-free for over six months. Many quit successfully only after several tries. Remember, too, that right now about forty-seven million Americans are former smokers who have quit. To successfully quit smoking, the American Cancer Society states that four factors are key:

- Making the decision to quit
- Setting a quit date and choosing a quit plan
- Dealing with withdrawal
- Staying quit (maintenance)

If you do lapse, don't give up. Just start again.

Blood Sugar and Diabetes

Diabetes mellitus is a group of conditions in which insulin production or processing is insufficient to absorb *glucose*, the body's main source of energy. It occurs in two forms. *Type I diabetes mellitus*, or insulin-dependent diabetes mellitus (once called juvenile-onset diabetes), usually has an abrupt onset in childhood or adolescence. It has a peak age of onset of twelve years, although it can develop at any age. Patients have an absolute lack of *insulin* in the body. Insulin is needed in order for the body to absorb glucose, and almost all patients with type I diabetes must take insulin injections in order to sustain life. Without insulin, diabetic ketoacidosis develops, which is characterized by vomiting; dehydration; deep, gasping breathing; confusion; and coma. Prior to the discovery of insulin in 1921 by Sir Frederick Banting and colleagues, diabetic ketoacidosis was a universally fatal disease.

Type II diabetes mellitus, or non-insulin-dependent diabetes mellitus (formerly called adult-onset or maturity-onset diabetes), develops more gradually. The early stages are characterized by *insulin resistance* or reduced insulin sensitivity (insulin becomes less effective at lowering glucose levels in the blood), accompanied by increased insulin production. At this stage, blood glucose levels can often be controlled through lifestyle adjustments, particularly diet and exercise. Medications may sometimes be necessary to improve insulin sensitivity or to reduce the production of glucose by the liver. If the disease worsens, the pancreas eventually becomes unable to produce sufficient insulin to maintain normal glucose levels. At this point, replacement of insulin with injections may be necessary in some patients. In the past, type II diabetes has generally occurred after adolescence, with a peak age of onset of fifty or sixty years. However, in recent years, type II has begun appearing increasingly in adolescents, due largely to an epidemic of childhood obesity.

Both types of diabetes significantly increase risk for microvascular (small blood vessel) and macrovascular (large blood vessel) complications. *Macrovascular complications* refer to cardiovascular disease of the large arteries that supply the heart, brain, and legs, while *microvascular complications* describe the small blood vessels that feed the eyes, kidneys, and nerves. In the days before insulin and oral therapy for diabetes, most people with diabetes died of causes such as coma, renal failure, and infection. Today, individuals with diabetes are two to four times more likely to die from heart disease than people without diabetes, and cardiovascular disease accounts for approximately two-thirds of deaths in diabetic patients.[39] Moreover, coronary heart disease occurs at an earlier age in people with diabetes. Diabetes also confers increased risk for microvascular disease, which can damage the eyes, resulting in loss of vision; kidneys, causing renal failure; or nerves, leading to numbness or pain throughout the body, often in the legs.

Why do people with diabetes have earlier and more atherosclerotic disease? In part, the additional risk can be attributed to the multiple major risk factors that characterize most cases of diabetes. Many individuals with diabetes also fit the criteria for *metabolic syndrome*, which is characterized by hypertension, an abnormal lipid profile, high glucose levels, inflammation, and increased blood clotting. The metabolic syndrome is strongly linked to obesity since obesity can cause all of the characteristics of the metabolic syndrome (see the section on obesity and the metabolic syndrome). A survey of the US population showed that 87 percent of adults older than fifty years who had diabetes also fit the criteria for the metabolic syndrome.[40] Approximately 80 percent of type II diabetes cases are related to obesity, and increasing numbers of children are developing diabetes due to obesity.

In addition, individuals with diabetes and metabolic syndrome are more likely to have a lipid profile that is associated with increased atherosclerosis.[41] The combination of elevated triglycerides, low HDL-C, and small dense LDL particles is a common problem in people with diabetes or the metabolic syndrome, and it is referred to as the lipid triad or atherogenic dyslipidemia. Small dense LDL particles are more susceptible to oxidation in the arterial wall, which means that they are more likely to cause damage to a blood vessel's inner surface and to become incorporated in a growing atherosclerotic lesion. Furthermore, researchers hypothesize that the elevated glucose levels and insulin resistance associated with diabetes may cause direct changes that accelerate atherosclerosis and increase the likelihood of developing cardiovascular disease. Elevated glucose levels and insulin resistance may constrict blood vessels and damage their inner lining, and they may promote the development of atherosclerotic lesions by increasing inflammation at the site of damage. Damage of the endothelium, or inner surface of a blood vessel, may in turn weaken the fibrous cap encasing atherosclerotic plaques, leaving them more prone to rupture.

Diabetes can be diagnosed using one of three measurements. The *fasting plasma glucose* (FPG) is a blood test that measures blood sugar levels after fasting for at least eight hours. People with levels that are at least 126 mg/dL (or 7.0 mmol/L) are diagnosed as having diabetes, while people with levels from 100 to 125 mg/dL (5.6–6.9 mmol/L) are considered to have *impaired fasting glucose* (IFG). The second test, *the oral glucose tolerance test* (OGTT), requires at least two blood samples. Blood is collected at the beginning of the test, and the patient is asked to drink a glucose solution. After two hours, blood is again drawn to determine how quickly the body clears glucose from the system. People with levels that are at least 200 mg/dL (11.1 mmol/L) are diagnosed as diabetic, while those with levels from 140 to 199 mg/dL (7.8–11.0 mmol/L) are considered to have *impaired glucose tolerance*. People with either impaired fasting glucose or impaired glucose tolerance are classified as having prediabetes. The third blood test measures glycated hemoglobin (also called glycosylated hemoglobin, hemoglobin A1c, or HbA_{1c}), a protein carried by red blood cells that has reacted with glucose in the blood, which provides an indication of average glucose levels during the preceding few months. Glycated hemoglobin levels at 6.5 percent or above indicate diabetes, while levels between 5.7 and 6.4 percent are considered prediabetes.

Prediabetes substantially increases risk for developing diabetes. Studies have found that the best way to prevent the development of diabetes is through lifestyle changes, including improved diet, increased exercise, and weight loss. Prediabetes is also considered to be an emerging risk factor for cardiovascular disease. It is currently unclear to what degree prediabetes increases cardiovascular risk, but an analysis of sixteen studies estimated a 20 percent increase in risk for heart disease with prediabetes.[42] If prediabetes progresses to diabetes, cardiovascular risk may further increase.

In individuals with diabetes, improved control of glucose levels has been shown to reduce the risk of microvascular complications, which can affect the small blood vessels of the eyes and kidneys and lead to nerve damage throughout the body. However, recent studies have not shown that tight glucose control reduces the risk of macrovascular complications, including cardiovascular disease. One of the authors (AMG) chaired the safety committee of a recent clinical trial called ACCORD, which tested the hypothesis that lowering glucose levels to near normal would reduce cardiovascular events in patients with diabetes.[43] However, this turned out not to be the case. The study included 10,250 diabetic patients with cardiovascular disease or additional cardiovascular risk factors who were either assigned to a standard-therapy group or an intensive-therapy group. Both groups received counseling and glucose-lowering medications and were asked to reduce their glycated hemoglobin (HbA$_{1c}$) levels; however, the intensive-therapy group had a much lower target (< 6 percent), close to that found in nondiabetic individuals (generally 3.5–5.5 percent). After three and a half years, 257 patients in the intensive-therapy group died compared to 203 patients in the standard-therapy group, which represents a statistically significant difference. In addition, intensive glucose lowering did not reduce the risk of suffering a cardiovascular event. Due to evidence of increased deaths with intensive therapy, this portion of the ACCORD trial was stopped. Two other recent clinical trials did not show an increase in the number of deaths with intensive glucose lowering, but neither did they show any cardiovascular benefit.[44] Thus, it appears that intensive glucose lowering does not reduce cardiovascular risk and might even be harmful in high-risk patients with diabetes, particularly those with long-standing diabetes. It is currently recommended that people with diabetes maintain Hb$_{A1c}$ levels between 7 and 7.5 percent.

Controlling your cardiovascular risk factors, including the diabetes itself, is very important if you have diabetes. Risk factor control includes a prescribed meal plan, exercise, weight control, and glucose control using oral medications or insulin. Diet is the cornerstone of treatment for diabetes and must be balanced with exercise and medication for optimal control of glucose. If you exercise heavily, more calories or less medication will be required. Weight loss is important if you are overweight. Glucose levels should be carefully monitored in all diabetic individuals. When blood sugar is tested before meals, it should be between 70 and 130 mg/dL; after meals, it should be < 180 mg/dL. Smoking, even smoking less than one pack of cigarettes per day, significantly increases risk for death from cardiovascular disease in people with diabetes, so make efforts to stop smoking as soon as possible.

In general, national guidelines recommend that risk factor goals be lower in diabetic patients because of their high risk. For example, people with diabetes are generally advised by their physicians to achieve lower LDL-C levels because their diabetes places them in the same risk category as people with a history of CHD. In terms of treatment for elevated LDL-C levels, people with diabetes have been shown to experience the same benefit from treatment with statins as nondiabetic patients.[45] Recently, statins have been shown to slightly increase the risk of developing diabetes, but in our opinion, this risk is far outweighed by the proven benefits of statin therapy, in both diabetic and nondiabetic patients (see the section on statins previously discussed in this chapter). Fibrates are another option in diabetic patients with low HDL-C and elevated triglycerides, but resins and nicotinic acid should not be used, as they have the potential to further increase triglycerides and insulin resistance.

Recently, some physicians have come upon an unexpected finding: bariatric surgery (weight-loss surgery) may provide an immediate improvement for diabetes. In very obese individuals, insulin and blood sugar levels have been shown to return to normal within a few days following bariatric surgery. Since these changes occur so quickly, it is unlikely that they are the result of weight loss due to the surgery. Some physicians hypothesize that bariatric surgery alters the anatomy of the small intestines, resulting in increased production of incretins, which are gastrointestinal hormones that increase insulin production.[46] While the use of surgery to treat type II diabetes remains controversial, researchers are continuing to gain insights within this emerging field.

Diet

Consuming a healthy diet throughout the life span is the best way to reduce cardiovascular risk and prevent the development of heart disease. A healthy diet can help you achieve and maintain desirable levels of total cholesterol and LDL-C, blood sugar, body weight, and blood pressure. Making dietary changes will be one of the first things your doctor will ask you to do if you have elevated cholesterol or other major cardiovascular risk factors. It is important that you follow through on these dietary recommendations for the rest of your life, even if you are eventually prescribed cholesterol-lowering medication. Consuming an unhealthy, fatty diet while taking these medications will cause them to work less effectively. In addition, deciding to adopt a healthier diet will leave you feeling and looking better than ever.

The American Heart Association recommends that instead of focusing on specific nutrients or food, individuals should try to consume an overall healthy diet (see table 2.7).[47] The AHA recommends eating a variety of fruits, vegetables, and grains, especially whole grains, in part because these foods are high in fiber. Fiber is associated with reduced cardiovascular risk. Deeply colored fruits and vegetables such as spinach, carrots, peaches, and berries are particularly encouraged because they tend to have more micronutrients than vegetables such as potatoes and corn. Choose low-fat or fat-free dairy products, and also include a variety of legumes, poultry, lean meat, and fish. Oily fish, such as salmon, trout, and mackerel, contain high amounts of omega-3 fatty acids, which are associated with decreased risk of death from heart disease. At least two servings of fish, at approximately eight ounces each, should be consumed each week. If you have coronary heart disease, try to consume approximately 1 gram of omega-3 fatty acids (EPA and DHA) per day, preferably from fish, although you may want to consider omega-3 dietary supplements in consultation with your physician. Fish such as canned light tuna, salmon, pollock, and catfish are generally lower in mercury content than shark, swordfish, king mackerel, and tilefish. Children and pregnant women should avoid eating fish with higher potential for mercury contamination. For middle-aged and older individuals, the benefits of regular fish consumption outweigh the potential risks of mercury contamination.

In addition to trying to improve overall eating habits, limit your consumption of saturated fat, *trans* fat, and dietary cholesterol, which are the three dietary components that significantly affect cholesterol levels in the blood.

Saturated fat, found in meats and certain plant oils, raises blood cholesterol. In the typical American diet, about two-thirds of the saturated fat consumed comes from animal products. These include butterfat (in butter, whole milk, cheese, cream, sour cream, and ice cream) and fat from meat (beef, pork, lamb, and poultry). Plant oils that are high in saturated fat are palm, coconut, and palm kernel oils. Saturated fat intake should be limited to less than 7 percent of total calories.

Trans fats are formed when vegetable oils are partially hydrogenated, which transforms them into semisolid fats with a long shelf life. *Trans* fats are often used commercially in deep-frying and baking, and they can be found in packaged snack foods, margarines, and crackers. *Trans* fats increase blood cholesterol, perhaps to a greater degree than saturated fat, and they also raise LDL-C and lower HDL-C levels. *Trans* fat intake should be limited to less than 1 percent of total calories. Substituting vegetable oils for partially hydrogenated fats can help reduce *trans* fat intake. Beginning in 2006, food manufacturers have been required to list *trans* fat content on package labels, so careful attention to this information should make it easier to monitor consumption. In addition, some large cities, beginning with New York City in 2007, have banned cooking with *trans* fat in restaurants.

Table 2.7. Making Healthy Food Choices[48]

- Balance calorie intake and exercise to maintain a healthy body weight.
  - o All adults should exercise at least 30 minutes a day on most days of the week.
- Limit your intake of saturated fat to <7% of energy, *trans* fat to <1% of energy, and cholesterol to <300 mg per day.
  - o Drink fat-free (skim) or low-fat dairy products.
  - o Cook fish, meat, and poultry by grilling, baking, or broiling and don't eat the skin on poultry.
  - o Cook with liquid vegetable oils instead of butter and margarine.
  - o Cut back on pastries, muffins, and donuts.
  - o Avoid deep-fried fast foods.
- Consume a diet rich in vegetables and fruits.
  - o Deeply colored vegetables and fruits (spinach, carrots, peaches, berries, etc.) tend to have more nutrients.
  - o Fruit juice is not the same as whole fruit.
- Choose whole-grain, high-fiber foods.
  - o Try whole wheat, oats/oatmeal, rye, barley, corn, popcorn, brown rice, wild rice, buckwheat, bulgur, millet, quinoa, and sorghum.
  - o Beans, fruits, and vegetables are also high in fiber.
- Consume fish, especially oily fish, at least twice a week.
  - o Canned light tuna, salmon, pollock, and catfish are lower in mercury than shark, swordfish, king mackerel, and tilefish.
- Minimize your intake of beverages and foods with added sugars.
- Reduce salt consumption.
  - o Cut back on condiments and processed meats.
  - o If you drink alcohol, do so in moderation.

Dietary cholesterol has variable effects on blood cholesterol levels in different people. There is a complicated relationship between the cholesterol you consume through food and the cholesterol that enters the bloodstream. Eating a high-cholesterol diet may not directly increase blood cholesterol levels in all individuals, but it may increase the ability of saturated fat to increase blood levels of cholesterol. Dietary cholesterol is found only in animal foods: egg yolk, meat, poultry, fish, and dairy products. Egg yolk is the most concentrated source of dietary cholesterol. People with heart disease should eat no more than two egg yolks per week. Egg whites, which do not contain cholesterol, can be consumed without limit. The AHA recommends that people with normal cholesterol levels consume less than 300 milligrams of cholesterol each day. If you already have elevated LDL-C levels, the NCEP recommends less than than 200 milligrams of cholesterol per day.

Reductions in saturated and *trans* fat and cholesterol can be achieved by selecting leaner meats and eating more fish and vegetables, by choosing fat-free or low-fat dairy products, and by avoiding commercially prepared fried and baked foods. Some people prefer a vegetarian approach, which can be equally satisfying and nutritious. In general, total fat intake can range between 25 and 35 percent, as long as saturated and *trans* fat consumption is kept low.

The AHA further recommends that calorie intake be balanced with physical activity in order to maintain a healthy body weight. To control calorie intake, individuals should read food labels to know how many calories they are actually consuming and also monitor portion size. Remember that fat-free foods can still be high in calories, as well as high in sugar. In general, Americans now consume large amounts of beverages and foods with added sugars (sucrose, corn syrup, and high-fructose corn syrup). Non-diet soft drinks, for example, contain a lot of added sugars and provide few nutrients, and excess consumption can quickly lead to weight gain. Try to minimize the amount of food with added sugars that you eat. Also try to limit sodium intake in order to keep blood pressure levels low (see the hypertension section previously discussed in this chapter).

In some studies, moderate alcohol consumption has been linked to decreased cardiovascular risk, although researchers are not entirely sure how or why this is so. A lot of media attention has been paid to red wine, but other alcoholic beverages may have a similar beneficial effect. Moderate alcohol consumption has been shown to modestly increase HDL-C levels. Despite these potential benefits, alcohol consumption is also associated with significant health risks, so it is not recommended that nondrinkers begin drinking to try to improve their cardiovascular health. If you do drink, limit alcohol intake to two drinks per day for men and one drink per day for women. One drink is equal to 0.5 ounce or 15 milliliters of ethanol (12 ounces of beer, 5 ounces of wine, or 1.5 ounces of eighty-proof whiskey).

Obesity and the Metabolic Syndrome

Obesity, which results from excessive calorie intake, is defined as having a body mass index (BMI) of 30 kg/m^2 or higher, while people are considered overweight if their BMI is between 25 and 30 kg/m^2. A desirable and healthy BMI is between 18.5 and 24.9 kg/m^2. The National Heart, Lung, and Blood Institute website (http://www.nhlbisupport.com/bmi/) provides an online BMI calculator, where you can enter your height and weight using either standard or metric measures.

Currently, about one-third of American adults are obese, and an additional one-third are overweight. The prevalence of obesity has increased dramatically over the past three decades. If this trend continues, it is estimated that by 2015, 41 percent will be obese, and an additional 34 percent will be overweight.[49] Obesity and obesity-related diseases are associated with race, with African Americans and Hispanic Americans experiencing greater rates of both compared to white Americans. Unfortunately, children and adolescents share the burden of obesity. In the United States, approximately nine million children between the ages of six and nineteen years are considered overweight, and approximately 70 percent of overweight adolescents will go on to become overweight adults.[50] The percentage of overweight children is also increasing, from approximately 6 percent in the early 1970s to 18 percent in 2007–2008.

Obesity and overweight are associated with decreased life expectancy. Forty-year-old nonsmoking men and women who are overweight have an estimated decrease in life expectancy of three years, while their counterparts who are obese can be expected to live six to seven years less than nonobese individuals.[51] Some of the medical hazards associated with obesity include an increased risk for heart disease, diabetes, and hypertension, as well as non-cardiovascular related conditions such as obstructive sleep apnea, gallbladder disease, some cancers, arthritis, orthopedic complications, and mood disorders.

Obesity exacerbates cardiovascular risk factors. It can raise the levels of blood cholesterol, triglycerides, blood pressure, and blood sugar and can lower the level of HDL-C. Obesity is a primary component of the metabolic syndrome, which is a group of risk factors that commonly occur together and greatly increase cardiovascular risk. The risk factors that make up the metabolic syndrome include abdominal obesity, elevated triglycerides and low HDL-C, hypertension, and elevated blood sugar (see table 2.8). Abdominal, or central, obesity is associated with an "apple" body type, as compared to a "pear" shape, and is more closely linked to increased cardiovascular risk than fat that accumulates around the hips and buttocks. The metabolic syndrome is also characterized by chronic inflammation and a tendency for increased blood clotting. It is believed that when fat cells increase in size, they release inflammatory molecules. As a result, fat is characterized by a chronic state of inflammation, which as we discussed in the previous chapter, is particularly conducive to the growth of atherosclerotic plaques. This chronic inflammation may help explain why obese individuals are at increased risk for heart disease.

Table 2.8. Metabolic Syndrome Risk Factors[52]

The presence of three or more of the following qualifies as metabolic syndrome:

- Abdominal obesity (waist circumference >40 inches in men, >35 inches in women)
- Triglycerides ≥ 150 mg/dL
- Low HDL-C (<40 mg/dL in men, <50 mg/dL in women)
- Blood pressure ≥130/≥85 mm Hg
- Fasting plasma glucose (FPG) ≥110 mg/dL

Weight loss can help lower cholesterol levels, blood pressure, and blood glucose. In order to control these cardiovascular risk factors, it is important to maintain a healthy body weight. If you are overweight or obese, try for a weight loss of 5 to 10 percent of your initial body weight. Many people need to reduce calorie consumption by five hundred to one thousand calories per day so that weight loss occurs at a rate of one to two pounds per week. Studies show that this moderate degree of weight loss will decrease your chances of developing diabetes by more than half, and it will substantially improve your other risk factors.

Weight loss is best achieved and sustained by combining a low-fat diet, regular aerobic exercise, and counseling. Counseling might include participating in programs such as Weight Watchers®, meeting with a nutritionist or dietician, or joining a support group. Recently there has been increased interest in weight-loss-counseling programs via telephone. Such programs have been found to be as effective as face-to-face counseling in helping people to lose weight, and they can be more convenient and less expensive, particularly for people living outside urban areas.

If you are obese and are having difficulty losing weight with diet and exercise, you might want to consider weight-loss medications. There are currently only a few weight-loss drugs that have been approved by the FDA, including orlistat (Xenical®, Alli®) and phentermine. Another drug, sibutramine (Meridia®), was withdrawn from the market in the United States after it was found to increase the risk for heart attack and stroke.[53] In general, the amount of weight lost with orlistat and phentermine is about 5 to 10 percent greater than the amount generally lost through diet and exercise alone. There are many other weight-loss products available over the counter, but these are not FDA approved and are considered dietary supplements. Dietary supplements are not regulated, so there is no medical evidence that they are safe or effective. You should consult a physician or registered dietician if you are considering taking a dietary supplement or would like to discuss the option of prescription weight-loss medication.

Orlistat is available in prescription form as Xenical and over the counter as Alli. The prescription version contains twice the dose of the over-the-counter version. Orlistat works by blocking the absorption of fat in the gastrointestinal tract. Common side effects are gastrointestinal and include fatty stools, oily diarrhea, and gas, which result because fat in the diet is not being absorbed. Consuming a high-fat diet while taking orlistat will result in gastrointestinal side effects, so patients must be committed to substantially reducing their fat intake while on this medication in particular. Orlistat may also block the absorption of nutrients in the body, so taking a multivitamin at a different time than the orlistat is recommended.

Phentermine is generic and is the least expensive and most widely used of the weight-loss medications. It is similar to amphetamines, and it suppresses the appetite by stimulating the release of the neurotransmitter norepinephrine in the brain. It is approved for short-term use only (generally up to twelve weeks). Phentermine was part of the popular Fen-Phen drug combination until 1997 when it was discovered that Fen-Phen increased the risk for heart valve disease. Fen-Phen was withdrawn from the market, but phentermine remains in use. Side effects may include depression, insomnia, increased blood pressure, irritability, and nervousness.

Psychosocial Factors

Psychosocial factors such as mental stress have long been linked with heart disease in the popular imagination. Only in the past few decades has scientific evidence to support this relationship begun to accumulate.[54] While it is now clear that psychosocial factors can play a role in the development of heart disease, it is more difficult to measure stress or anger, for example, than it is to measure cholesterol levels or blood pressure. Stress and emotions are very individual, and what disturbs one person may not bother another. Thus, researchers have not been able to demonstrate conclusively that psychosocial factors are risk factors for the development of atherosclerotic heart disease in the same way that high cholesterol or smoking are. In addition, there are very few clinical trials testing whether interventions such as counseling, psychotherapy, or antidepressants can improve survival following a cardiac event. With continuing research in this area, we expect to learn more about how our thinking and emotions affect our cardiovascular health.

Current research does indicate that depression, anxiety, stress, or anger can worsen an individual's heart disease and make recovery more difficult. In addition, stressful events and intense emotions are capable of triggering a coronary event such as angina, heart attack, or sudden cardiac death in some individuals.

The strongest data show a relation between depression and coronary heart disease. Studies indicate that people with depression are at higher risk for developing new heart disease and for having recurrent events if they have already been diagnosed with heart disease. Patients with coronary heart disease are also more likely to be depressed compared to people without heart disease, in large part due to the effects of their illness. Other factors including social isolation and occupational stress have also been associated with increased risk for heart disease. Being married or having a close friend or confidant, for example, has been shown to reduce cardiovascular risk and to increase survival following a heart attack. Some research suggests that Monday mornings are the most common time for heart attacks, possibly because the return to work can cause a sharp increase in blood pressure in some individuals. Studies regarding the relationship between heart disease and anger, hostile behavior, aggressiveness, and anxiety have been mixed, with some showing increased cardiovascular risk for individuals with one or more of these traits while others do not.

Most people have heard of the type A personality, which was initially described more than fifty years ago and is characterized by competitiveness, time urgency (a feeling of being pressured or rushed), and aggression. For several decades, much research has examined the relation between type A personality and heart disease, but results have been inconclusive. In recent years, the concept of the type A personality has been criticized by many in the medical and scientific community as being obsolete. Attention has shifted instead to the so-called type D ("distressed") personality, which is characterized by negative emotions such as worry, anxiety, and pessimism and by emotional and social inhibition. Type D personality is similar to depression, except that it describes a chronic tendency toward experiencing negative emotions rather than isolated episodes of depression. Studies suggest that heart disease patients with type D personality are at increased risk for future cardiovascular problems compared to other patients, although evidence in this field is still preliminary and evolving.

Psychosocial factors may negatively impact cardiovascular health by affecting an individual's behavior. For example, stress can indirectly increase risk for heart disease by causing people to smoke, overeat, drink excessively, or stop exercising. Smoking, eating a diet high in fat, drinking too much alcohol, having a physically inactive lifestyle, and being obese then each directly increase a person's risk for developing heart disease. Similarly, someone who is depressed or socially isolated may avoid going to the doctor or be neglectful about taking prescribed medications.

It is also hypothesized that psychosocial factors like long-term stress can have a negative effect on the body's normal functioning, which can then play a role in the development of heart disease. Long-term stress can weaken the immune system and leave some people more vulnerable to colds or infections. It may confer an increased risk for high blood pressure, particularly in men. Theories have proposed that stress may also increase risk for heart disease by making the heart pump harder and faster, by altering heart rhythms, by causing the blood to become stickier, and by increasing inflammation within the bloodstream and blood vessel wall. These effects may make it more likely that a person with underlying atherosclerosis may develop symptoms of heart disease or experience a coronary event.

Another role that psychosocial factors might play in heart disease is as a trigger of acute events such as angina, heart attack, or sudden cardiac death. The eighteenth-century anatomist and surgeon Dr. John Hunter understood that emotional fervor can bring on painful chest pains and one day died suddenly, collapsing after a dispute with colleagues. He had earlier predicted the manner of his own death, saying that his life, because of his angina and temper, was at the mercy of any rascal who chose to upset him.[55]

Studies have sought to make sense of the link between stressful events and cardiovascular events. One study, for example, found risk for having a heart attack to be more than doubled during the two hours after an episode of anger.[56] On January 17, 1994, the day of the Northridge, California, earthquake, there was a sharp increase in the number of sudden cardiac deaths in Los Angeles County: twenty-four deaths, as opposed to a daily average of 4.6 deaths during the week preceding the earthquake.[57] Only three of the twenty-four deaths were related to unusual physical exertion. Similarly, sudden cardiac deaths increased among the Israeli civilian population during the first ten days of the Gulf War in 1991.[58] Some, but not all, studies found that the September 11, 2001, attacks on the World Trade Center were associated with an increased risk for heart attacks on the days immediately following. Sporting events and deer hunting have also been associated with increased cardiovascular risk.

How extreme stress might lead to a cardiac event is complex, but it may involve an increased demand by the heart muscle for oxygen due to an increased heart rate and blood pressure. If the heart's demand for oxygen is not met, the result may be the chest pain of angina, or part of the heart muscle may die (a heart attack). Like strenuous physical activity, mental stress may also cause atherosclerotic plaques to rupture, which can lead to the formation of blood clots and a resulting heart attack or stroke. Stress may be more likely to trigger a coronary event in people who have already developed atherosclerosis within their arteries, whether or not they have had prior systems of heart disease. One study examined forty-three cases of stress-related sudden death.[59] The stress was fear in fifteen cases, an altercation in twenty-one cases, sexual activity in three cases, and police questioning or arrest in four cases. Subjects ranged in age from twenty to ninety-two years. Thirty-eight of the deaths were due to cardiac causes, and twenty-seven of those to atherosclerotic heart disease. Autopsy findings led the investigators to conclude that stress-related sudden death occurs primarily in individuals with severe underlying heart disease, especially atherosclerotic heart disease.

A severely stressful episode can also trigger an arrhythmia (irregular heartbeat) or a disturbance of the heart's electrical stability, which can lead to sudden death. When the body is faced with an acute stressor, a "fight-or-flight" response is activated. Stress hormones are released to organize the heart and lungs, as well as the circulation, metabolism, and immune systems, to deal immediately with the threat. These hormones cause the heart rate to speed up, which can trigger a fatal arrhythmia in susceptible individuals (see chapter 6 for more on arrhythmias).

It is important to remember that stress is not inherently negative. Rather, it's how individual people cope with the stress in their lives that determines whether or not it ends up negatively affecting their cardiovascular health. Some people are highly tolerant of stress, while others can be very sensitive to stress. Although most people experience significant stress at some point in their lives, not everyone develops physical problems because of it. The less control people have over stressful situations and the more uncertainty they feel as a result, the more likely they are to experience the negative effects of stress. Someone who has more than one chronic stressor that is not easily controlled, such as a high-pressure job, aging parents, and an unhappy family life, may be more likely to develop stress-related health problems. Personality traits, such as being neurotic, generally anxious, or prone to addictive behaviors, may increase the stress response in some people. Outgoing people may tend to become less stressed out. Genetic factors or the impact of one's childhood can also make someone more or less likely to respond negatively to a stressful situation. People lacking a social network may find it difficult to relieve their stress if they are unable to talk about it with others.

Some of the best ways to relieve stress are by making lifestyle changes. Exercising regularly, eating a healthy diet, stopping smoking, and avoiding excessive alcohol and caffeine consumption can both improve your overall health and improve your resistance to stress. Deep breathing from the diaphragm, which increases the amount of oxygen in your lungs; muscle-relaxing exercises, in which you systematically focus on relaxing different sets of muscles throughout your body; and meditation, which focuses your mind on a positive thought and away from everyday worries, all help your body relax. Meditation, exercise, and psychotherapy are three techniques that many people have found useful for managing stress.

Meditation is learning how to stop everything you are doing and start paying attention to the present moment. It is learning how to make time for yourself, how to slow down and nurture calmness and self-acceptance, and how to observe what your mind is up to from moment to moment. It is simply being present—not living in the past or future, just paying attention to the present. The more regularly you practice meditation, the more it will work for you. A successful way to start meditating is to concentrate on your breathing—the air as it goes in and out of your nose. When learning to meditate, most students find it helpful to have a teacher.

Exercise also fulfills the requirement of focusing the mind outside everyday worries, and it relaxes the body by stretching muscles. Of course, with exercise you get the added benefit of an improved physical condition (see the section in this chapter on physical activity). Exercise has also been proven to be an effective treatment for depression, and it helps improve self-esteem, wards off feelings of anxiety, and reduces stress.

You may also want to consider counseling or psychotherapy to help with stress management or feelings of depression or anxiety. It may be particularly helpful to enlist support if you have recently been diagnosed with heart disease or have suffered a cardiac event. Often counseling is a component of cardiac rehabilitation programs (see chapter 5). A 2011 study conducted at Uppsala University Hospital in Sweden found that psychotherapy can help prevent recurrent cardiac events.[60] The study compared group-cognitive-behavioral therapy with standard medical treatment in 362 people who had suffered a heart attack or had coronary artery bypass surgery. The group-therapy participants were taught how to reduce stress in their lives. After two years, people who had received group therapy had 45 percent fewer heart attacks than those who had received medication, and they were less likely to have died from a cardiac cause. If you feel like you might benefit from psychotherapy or counseling, you may want to consider asking your cardiologist or primary care doctor for a referral.

Physical Inactivity

Americans are becoming an increasingly sedentary population. In 2008–2009, 32 percent of adults engaged in regular leisure-time physical activity, while 33 percent engaged in no leisure-time physical activity.[61] Children are also engaging in less exercise and are instead playing more video games and watching more television. Only 57 percent of male adolescents and 40 percent of female adolescents aged fourteen to seventeen meet currently recommended levels of physical activity.

According to the American Heart Association, people who are physically inactive are 1.5 to 2.4 times more likely to develop coronary heart disease.[62] This increased risk is equivalent to the risk experienced by people with high cholesterol or hypertension or those who smoke. Regular moderate exercise, which can entail something as easy and inexpensive as brisk walking, provides a wealth of benefits to your health. Regular exercise can reduce the risk for heart disease, stroke, diabetes, arthritis, osteoporosis, and colon cancer. It can lower blood pressure, improve circulation and digestion, and increase energy. It helps control blood sugar levels in the body, thus preventing the development of diabetes. It improves the lipid profile by increasing HDL-C and by lowering LDL-C and triglyceride levels. In addition to increasing calorie expenditure, exercise helps with weight control by naturally curbing the appetite. It also has psychological benefits, including relief of anxiety and improvement of mood, concentration, alertness, and productivity. Exercise strengthens muscles and can improve an individual's sense of well being, self-esteem, and body image.

Exercise reduces the risk for coronary heart disease both directly and indirectly. Aerobic exercise improves cardiovascular fitness by getting the heart pumping and causing it to become more efficient. It protects the inner lining of blood vessels (endothelium) by keeping vessels flexible and less prone to developing atherosclerosis. Exercise reduces cardiovascular risk indirectly through its effects on risk factors. By helping to control body weight, blood pressure, cholesterol, and blood sugar levels, exercise has a positive effect on all aspects of the metabolic syndrome, thereby decreasing overall risk.

Another important benefit of regular exercise is that it reduces the risk that strenuous exercise may trigger a heart attack or sudden cardiac death. Sudden, vigorous activity by people who are unaccustomed to it can be dangerous. The temporary risk period is the time spent exercising and about one hour afterward, a period that may account for about one in twenty heart attacks (some studies have shown as many as one in ten). The reasons behind this phenomenon are not fully understood, but it is believed that exercise may disrupt atherosclerotic plaques. Also, in sedentary people, but not active people, strenuous activity leads to changes in platelet activity that could contribute to or initiate thrombosis (the formation of blood clots). The excess risk associated with vigorous exercise decreases as your level of physical activity increases.

Evidence shows that only moderate exercise is required to achieve health benefits. Ideally, individuals should exercise throughout their entire lives. Experts recommend that everyone should engage in moderate physical activity for thirty minutes or more on most, and preferably all, days of the week. Individuals who are trying to lose weight should exercise for at least one hour on most days of the week. It is possible to become moderately fit in only ten weeks through engaging in activities such as the following on most days of the week: thirty minutes of brisk walking; fifteen minutes of jogging; thirty minutes of lawn mowing, raking, or gardening; or bicycling three miles in thirty minutes. The activity does not need to be performed all at once in order to achieve benefit. What is important is the total amount of activity performed, so it can be ten minutes here and ten minutes there. Incorporating moderate exercise into your daily routine can be as simple as taking the stairs instead of the elevator or parking a little farther away from your destination and walking the remainder of the trip.

Experts additionally recommend that all adults engage in activities that promote muscular strength or endurance on at least two days a week. Resistance or strength training helps build strong bones and prevents bone loss in middle age, thus decreasing the risk for osteoporosis. Increased muscle mass increases the body's metabolism, which can help with weight control. Increased muscular strength and endurance is also associated with increased longevity.

Before beginning an exercise regimen, be sure to talk to your physician. Also, make sure to begin any program of increased physical activity gradually. While the risk for heart attack or sudden cardiac death from physical exertion is relatively low in the population as a whole, it can be high for any given individual. People who are at high risk for coronary heart disease or who have a history of coronary heart disease may be asked to undergo exercise electrocardiography (ECG) to establish a suitable level of exercise (see chapter 3). If you plan to use heart rate to measure the intensity of your exercise, also talk with your physician about your recommended target heart rate during exercise.

Types of Exercise

Before beginning your exercise program, you should decide on an overall goal. Consider whether you want to lose weight, increase endurance and stamina, strengthen your muscles, or gain flexibility. You may want a combination of all of the above. After determining what effect you want to achieve, begin your workout by warming up (by walking, for instance). Exercise until you arrive at a level that requires just a little more effort than is comfortable, and then cool down. To ensure improvement, increase the number of times you exercise per week, exercise for a longer period each time, or increase the intensity of the exercise. However, never push yourself until you experience joint pain or chest pain.

Endurance Exercises

Endurance exercises build stamina and burn calories, both during the exercise and for a period of time after exercise is completed. These exercises employ large muscles such as those in the hips and legs in continuous motion at a moderate intensity for twenty to sixty minutes. Walking briskly outdoors or on a treadmill, hiking, jogging, outdoor or indoor cycling, swimming, rowing, using elliptical or stair-climbing machines, taking aerobic or step classes, cross-country skiing, and playing sports such as soccer and tennis all build endurance. While working out at a moderate intensity, you burn both oxygen and fuel (from the food you have eaten in the last three to eight hours and/or body fat) to produce energy for prolonged muscle contraction. You should not be exercising so intensely that you feel breathless or unable to talk. Aerobic endurance exercises are especially useful in cardiovascular conditioning and increase the strength and efficiency of the heart.

Strength Training

Strength training includes activities such as weight lifting, sit-ups, push-ups, and other body-lifting exercises. Each exercise builds specific muscles by working them briefly but intensely. If your goal is to build muscle mass, use heavier weights and few repetitions. If your goal is to strengthen and tone muscles, use lighter weights and more repetitions. As a starting point, choose a weight that you can lift comfortably for eight to twelve repetitions, but that leaves you feeling fatigued by the end of the set. Perform eight to ten different exercises per workout, and be sure to include all major muscle groups. You can choose to work out all muscle groups each time you exercise, or you can alternate between muscle groups on different days of the week (upper body and lower body, for instance).

Flexibility Exercises

Flexibility exercises, including yoga, enable your body's joints to move through a wider range of motion. The basic movement is to extend the muscle, hold it in position until light to moderate tension develops, and then continue the stretch for about ten seconds. Flexibility exercises should be done slowly and evenly. Do not bounce or push too hard when the muscle is extended or you could cause small tears in muscles and ligaments.

Warm-Up and Cool-Down

Whatever routine you choose, remember to allow your body time to warm up beforehand and cool down afterward. Try walking or gentle stretching (not bouncing) as a warm-up. Warm-up exercises gradually introduce activity, allowing the entire body to get properly ready for physical effort. Cool-down exercises, which might also include walking or stretching, alert your body's circulation and metabolism to return to a less active state.

Targeting Your Heart Rate

Building aerobic fitness increases your cardiovascular fitness. The intensity of a workout is sometimes measured by comparing your heart rate (pulse count) during exercise with a target exercise heart rate. Your maximum heart rate is determined by subtracting your age from 220. Never attempt to reach your maximum heart rate. Your target exercise heart rate is determined by multiplying your maximum heart rate by an appropriate percentage based on your level of fitness. Beginners should start out by trying to achieve 50 percent of their maximum heart rate. As your level of cardiovascular fitness increases, you can begin to increase your exercise intensity and corresponding target heart rate up to about 75 percent of your maximum heart rate.

Other Risk Factors

More than 250 risk factors for coronary heart disease have been described in scientific literature. Major risk factors have been scientifically proven to increase cardiovascular risk. Modification of a major risk factor, either through lifestyle changes or medication, has been shown to decrease risk for heart disease. New or emerging risk factors lack this level of proof. Evidence about an emerging risk factor may be contradictory, or measurement of the risk factor (often through blood tests) may not be standardized or easily available. Some of the measures discussed in the section in this chapter on lipids are considered emerging risk factors, including apolipoprotein B, non-HDL-C, LDL and HDL particle number and size, lipoprotein(a), apo B/apo A-I ratio, and TC/HDL-C ratio. In addition, prediabetes, which is defined as having impaired glucose tolerance or impaired fasting glucose, is an emerging risk factor for cardiovascular disease. Some experts consider psychosocial factors like stress to be an emerging risk factor until further data emerge. The evidence surrounding alcohol and heart disease is also somewhat contradictory since alcohol can increase blood pressure and lead to other health problems, while moderate drinking has been shown to decrease the risk for heart disease.

Physicians may find that measurements of emerging risk factors may be helpful in determining your overall cardiovascular risk and in deciding upon a course of preventive treatment. This section discusses just a few of the most well-researched emerging risk factors.

C-Reactive Protein

As we discussed in the previous chapter, C-reactive protein (CRP) is a marker of chronic inflammation in the body that has been consistently linked to increased cardiovascular risk in men and women. Results from the recent JUPITER trial indicate that patients who achieved the lowest levels of CRP and LDL-C experienced the greatest decrease in cardiovascular risk. Many heart attacks occur in healthy, middle-aged individuals, and measures of CRP can help doctors identify individuals who are at increased cardiovascular risk despite having relatively low levels of LDL-C. These at-risk patients may benefit from treatment with statins if their CRP levels are high.

Currently there are no guidelines regarding optimal CRP levels. CRP levels greater than 2 mg/L are generally considered elevated. Based on the results of JUPITER and other primary and secondary prevention trials, it appears that individuals who obtain CRP levels less than 1 mg/L, combined with LDL-C levels less than 70 mg/dL, are the least likely to experience a coronary event. Statins have been shown to lower CRP levels to varying degrees. Losing weight, exercising, and stopping smoking also reduce CRP levels, and you should try these lifestyle changes first if your CRP levels are elevated.

Homocysteine

An elevation of homocysteine, an amino acid, can damage muscles and predispose factors in the blood to form clots. As many as one-third of people with atherosclerosis have elevated blood levels of homocysteine. Major studies such as the Framingham Heart Study and the Physicians' Health Study have linked elevated levels of homocysteine with increased risk for heart attack and stroke.[63] Homocysteine is normally found in very small amounts in the blood (about 1/1000 of the concentration of cholesterol), and risk appears to increase if levels are elevated by 20 to 30 percent.

Elevated levels of homocysteine are caused by deficiencies in folic acid, vitamin B_6, and vitamin B_{12}. For many years, scientists hypothesized that reducing levels of homocysteine by taking supplements of folic acid or vitamin B would reduce CHD risk. However, several recent clinical trials have demonstrated that this is not the case, and reducing levels of homocysteine has not been shown to reduce risk.[64] Although supplements are not recommended for the prevention of heart disease, folic acid remains important to a balanced diet. Rich sources include fortified oatmeal, wheat germ, spinach, broccoli, turnip greens, brussels sprouts, lettuce, oranges, cantaloupes, strawberries, and legumes.

Fibrinogen

The protein fibrinogen plays a role in the clotting process and is associated with inflammation. Beginning in the 1970s, elevated fibrinogen in the blood has been linked to increased risk for heart attack and stroke. It is believed that fibrinogen contributes to heart attack and stroke risk by making blood more likely to clot and by increasing the clumping of platelets in the blood.

Fibrinogen levels are higher in women, in smokers, in people with diabetes or hypertension, and in people who are obese or sedentary. It is thought that the major cardiovascular risk factors contribute collectively to elevated fibrinogen levels. The lifestyle change that is key to lowering fibrinogen levels is smoking cessation. Lesser effects are achieved by weight loss and increased physical activity. There are no drugs that specifically lower fibrinogen levels. In some studies, the lipid-lowering class of drug called fibrates has been shown to reduce fibrinogen, but others have shown increases.

COMPLEMENTARY AND ALTERNATIVE MEDICINE

Complementary and alternative medicine refers to treatments that are not considered to be part of conventional medical practice. Its long history and diverse traditions go beyond the scope of this book but include Hildegard of Bingen's medicine, homeopathy, and Chinese medicine (Dr. Wighard Strehlow and Dr. Henry J. Greten from Germany have conducted work in these areas). Many complementary approaches have not been tested in clinical trials, although the National Institutes of Health have established a National Center for Complementary and Alternative Medicine (http://nccam.nih.gov) to conduct and support research in this field. One recent finding suggests that red yeast rice, which naturally contains the same active ingredient as the statin drug lovastatin, could be an alternative cholesterol-lowering treatment for patients unable to take statins.[65]

***

In this chapter, we have discussed major and emerging risk factors for cardio-vascular disease. Some of the major risk factors cannot be changed, such as personal history of CHD, family history of premature CHD, sex, and age. Others can be modified by making healthy lifestyle choices or by taking medications if necessary; those that can be modified include lipid levels (high LDL-C, low HDL-C, high triglycerides), high blood pressure, cigarette smoking, diabetes, diet, obesity and the metabolic syndrome, psychosocial factors, and physical inactivity. In addition, we have considered some of the emerging risk factors. These have included measures related to the concentration of various lipoproteins in the blood (apolipoprotein B, non-HDL-C, LDL and HDL particle number and size, lipoprotein(a), apo B/apo A-I ratio, and TC/HDL-C ratio), measures of blood sugar, CRP, homocysteine, and fibrinogen.

Information on risk factors can help you win the battle against heart disease. By taking steps to control your risk factors and by adopting an overall healthy lifestyle, you can decrease the chances of suffering a future heart attack or stroke. The strategies to lower the risks that we have discussed in this chapter have been medically proven to work in rigorous clinical trials.

In the next chapter, we discuss the various noninvasive and invasive diag-nostic tests that can be used to determine your cardiac health.

CHAPTER 3

DETERMINING YOUR CARDIAC HEALTH

For many people, visiting the doctor can be a stressful experience. Visiting a cardiologist, or a specialist trained to treat disorders of the heart and circulatory system, can cause additional anxiety, particularly if you are already having symptoms or have been referred by a primary care physician, family practitioner, or other doctor. Such feelings are normal. However, by arming yourself with information and knowing what to expect in advance, you can make the experience as pleasant as possible. Doctors and other members of the health care team, including physician assistants, nurses, and technicians, are there to help you by diagnosing and treating whatever problem you may be having. If you are not having symptoms but your doctor has ordered tests, don't worry that there is something wrong with you. Most likely, your doctor is just trying to determine your risk for heart disease or decide if you might benefit from preventive medication. If you have any questions or concerns, just ask.

The noninvasive and invasive diagnostic tests discussed in this section carry minor risks. Any procedure that involves exposure to radiation, taking medication orally or through an intravenous (IV) needle, or penetrating the skin is associated with some risk. However, the benefits of taking the test and acquiring the information provided by it often outweigh the risks. You should consult with your doctor about these risks and any concerns you might have. Do not be intimidated by having to sign consent forms. The precautions that hospitals and physicians take are meant to ensure your safety and guarantee that you fully understand exactly what to expect with the procedure.

The radiation doses used in diagnostic x-rays and computed tomography (CT) scans are much lower than those used for the treatment of diseases such as

115

cancer, and moreover the risk of developing cancer from these diagnostic tests is relatively low. Advances in medical technology have minimized patients' exposure to radiation in diagnostic tests and have increased their speed and accuracy. Medical imaging in particular has developed substantially in recent years, resulting in exceptionally clear and detailed views of the heart and blood vessels. Larger hospital facilities are more likely to have the newest and most sophisticated technologies available, although the most expensive tests (not covered by insurance) are not routinely ordered and are used only in special circumstances.

THE MEDICAL HISTORY AND THE PHYSICAL EXAMINATION

Before ordering any tests, a doctor generally meets with you in an office examining room in order to obtain a medical history and to perform a physical examination. One of the most important parts of the physical exam isn't physical at all. It's when the patient talks and the doctor—or someone else on the health care team—listens. Communicate your problem as clearly as you can. Make sure that you answer the questions that are asked, but also convey additional information that you may want your health care providers to be aware of.

Describing the Symptoms

If you are experiencing symptoms, only you know exactly what they feel like. At times, it can be difficult describing your pain or discomfort, but it is important that you provide as much detail as possible. Doctors need to know where it hurts, the character of the pain, and other symptoms and signs that go along with the pain. One way to provide a clear and accurate description is to plan ahead: if possible, keep a symptom diary for several days before your examination and then take the diary to your appointment. To help you record information that is most helpful to the physician, consider the following symptoms that may be associated with heart disease.

Chest Pain

Chest pain can be a symptom of a number of conditions, including heart disease. Chest pain associated with heart disease is due to a lack of oxygen reaching the heart. It may be localized to one area of the chest, or it may spread out, at times radiating to the arm, neck, jaw, or back. The sensation may feel dull, aching, burning, tight, or crushing. Sometimes it may feel like indigestion. Note the duration and severity of the pain or discomfort. Chest pain associated with angina comes and goes (see chapter 4 for more on angina and other forms of atherosclerotic disease). It can be triggered by physical exertion, emotional stress, eating, or exposure to cold temperatures. It may be relieved by rest, warmth, or medication. **Pain that is severe and that lasts longer than twenty minutes may be a sign of a heart attack and is a medical emergency.** If chest pain is accompanied by symptoms such as nausea, sweating, dizziness, shortness of breath, or anxiety, call an ambulance (9-1-1) immediately.

Breathing Problems

Labored or difficult breathing is called *dyspnea* and is associated with a wide variety of diseases of the heart and lungs, as well as with anxiety. Shortness of breath may indicate that your heart is not pumping enough oxygen to your body. It may occur due to exercise, or it may become worse when you are lying down or after you have been asleep for a few hours.

Fatigue

Fatigue is a common symptom frequently encountered by doctors. Note if your fatigue has been getting worse, if you have had to stop engaging in particular activities due to fatigue, or if you feel fatigue during a particular time of day.

Palpitations

Heart palpitations can be associated with arrhythmias (irregular heart rhythms) but are also often linked to stress, anxiety, or caffeine consumption. The heartbeat may feel rapid, irregular, or pounding, or it may feel like your heart is stopping or skipping beats. Note what brings palpitations on and if it is accompanied by other symptoms.

Leg Pain

Leg pain may be a sign of poor circulation resulting from peripheral artery disease, which is atherosclerosis that has developed in the arteries in the leg. Pain may occur in your foot, calf, thigh, or buttock, and it may be brought on by walking or other activity. Note whether pain is relieved by resting with your legs up or by keeping them down. Cramps in the legs at night, sometimes called "charley horses," are not a sign of peripheral artery disease. Pain that occurs at rest or that is burning, tingling, or numbing may indicate that your legs are receiving a critical lack of oxygen.

Fainting

Fainting is called *syncope* and usually results when there is insufficient blood flow to the brain. It may occur after strenuous physical activity.

Past Medical Profile and Risk Factors

In trying to construct an overall picture of you and arrive at a diagnosis, the doctor will inquire about your past medical history, risk factors, and lifestyle. Before your visit, it can be helpful to jot down injuries, hospitalizations, surgeries, pregnancies, recent dental procedures, past and present illnesses, and any allergies. Make a list of all the drugs you take now or have taken recently, and include the dosage and how often you take each one. (Alternatively, you can bring the containers with you.) The list should include both prescription and over-the-counter drugs such as painkillers, cold remedies, antacids, sleeping aids, vitamin or mineral supplements, herbal remedies, and any recreational or "street" drugs.

A family history of hypertension, heart disease, high blood cholesterol, stroke, or diabetes will let your physician know that you may be at risk of having one of these disorders. Your doctor will also ask questions regarding lifestyle: your usual pattern of diet and exercise, any recent change in your weight, past or present use of tobacco, intake of alcohol and caffeine, and sleep patterns, among others. If you are uncomfortable with a question, ask why it is needed.

Physical Exam

You may already be familiar with having your blood pressure and pulse measured. In a routine examination, the wrist is often the only place a pulse is assessed. The cardiologist may take your pulse at additional locations, such as inside the elbow, behind the knee, near the groin, behind the ankle, and on top of the foot, to see if the pulse varies at different places (see figure 3.1). To evaluate your heart, the doctor may feel or tap your chest, and she will listen to your heart and lungs with a stethoscope. The physician will observe the blood vessels in the eyes and feel and listen for signs of an abdominal aortic aneurysm (ballooning of the part of the aorta located in the abdomen).

A stethoscope may be used to detect blockages in the major arteries. Normally, blood flow through healthy arteries and veins is silent, but when there is an obstruction, a sound called a *bruit* (pronounced BREW-ee) can often be heard. Bruits are caused by turbulent blood flow and often indicate the presence of atherosclerosis. The two major blood vessels in the neck—the carotid arteries and the jugular veins—are of special interest. When the carotid artery is more than 30 to 40 percent obstructed, a bruit may be heard. Veins do not usually pulsate, but pressure changes in the right side of the heart can cause the jugular veins to pulsate. For this reason, the jugular pulse is a quick way to evaluate how well the right side of the heart is functioning. The jugular pulse is seen just above the collarbone but generally only when a person reclines, with shoulders propped up at about a forty-five-degree angle.

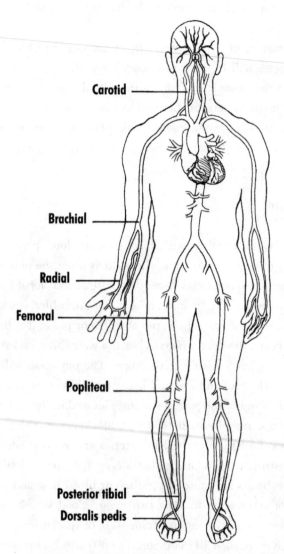

Figure 3.1. The seven sites at which the pulse can be easily felt on the human body. *Illustration created by Herbert R. Smith Jr.*

The physician may briefly examine your skin and nails and evaluate your skin's color, elasticity, temperature, and moisture. Normally skin is warm and dry, and the temperature is about the same in all parts of the body. A bluish tinge to the skin or nails, called *cyanosis*, can be a sign of poor oxygen supply in the blood. Long-standing cyanosis changes the shape of fingertips and nails. The fingers look bulbous, like clubs; nails flatten out; and the skin at the bottom of the nail bulges. In addition, peripheral artery disease can cause pitting, dents, brittleness, and thinning of the nails.

Peripheral artery disease usually involves the feet or legs, but occasionally the upper extremities are affected. To test circulation in the legs, the doctor will observe your skin, check your pulses, and may raise your legs to see if there is a change in color. Poor circulation can eventually cause hair loss on the extremity and skin that is thin, shiny, and smooth. If blood return to the heart is slowed down, the extremity may itch, look red and scaly, and develop brown spots. Varicose veins bulge when patients sit or stand, but when the legs are lifted above the heart, the veins look normal.

If you have any swelling in the lower legs, the doctor will try to determine how severe it is. Swelling can be a sign of *edema*, or too much fluid in the tissues. Edema can be caused by heart failure or by a blood clot or infection. To test for *pitting edema*, the doctor presses a finger against the shin or ankle for several seconds to see if it leaves an indentation and, if it does, for how long. *Non-pitting edema*, which is much less common, may have other causes such as hyperthyroidism (overactive thyroid gland). Swelling in the legs can also be caused by slow blood flow in the legs due to extended periods of immobility, such as a long airplane flight or prolonged bed rest.

Some blood tests a cardiologist might order, such as a lipid profile or tests for C-reactive protein (discussed in chapter 2), are used to determine your risk of developing heart disease in the future. If your physician suspects that you may already have heart disease, tests measuring *cardiac enzymes* (including troponin and creatine kinase), brain natriuretic peptide, and prothrombin might be ordered. Routine blood tests such as a *complete blood count* and a *comprehensive metabolic panel* may also be included. The complete blood count can help diagnose anemia, infections, allergies, and problems with blood cells and blood clotting. The comprehensive metabolic panel checks blood sugar (glucose) levels, electrolyte and fluid balance, and liver and kidney function.

NONINVASIVE DIAGNOSTIC PROCEDURES

Many heart problems can be diagnosed with tests that are noninvasive, which means that the procedure does not require penetrating the body. The noninvasive tests discussed below are safe, rarely cause discomfort, and seldom have side effects. They are generally less expensive than invasive tests. Some tests will probably be performed in your doctor's office, while others may be done at a hospital or other facility. If you feel nervous because you do not know what to expect—or if you are simply curious—ask the technician to explain the machine and test. Test results will be conveyed to you by your cardiologist or primary care physician.

Chest x-rays and electrocardiography (ECG) are both common tests that can be ordered for many reasons, including as part of a routine physical exam and as preparation before hospitalization or surgery. Chest x-rays can be used to monitor the heart's size and condition across time and can suggest the presence of conditions such as heart failure, although additional tests are usually necessary. ECG is the primary tool for diagnosing arrhythmias and is used to monitor patients in the hospital. It can establish whether a person is currently undergoing or has experienced a heart attack, and it may be used to determine whether a person with symptoms of heart disease may require further testing. Ambulatory ECG is generally conducted in people with suspected arrhythmias who require extended monitoring. Exercise stress testing can help diagnose heart disease in patients experiencing symptoms; those with positive results may be recommended for cardiac catheterization, or for CT or magnetic resonance angiography. Sometimes a physician may order a simple treadmill test using ECG to rule out coronary heart disease in a low-risk individual. Stress tests incorporating echocardiography, nuclear imaging, or MI are more accurate and may be ordered as a follow-up to exercise testing with an ECG. Exercise stress tests are also used to evaluate the effects of treatment and ability to exercise in patients with known heart disease.

Echocardiography is ordered when a patient has signs or symptoms of cardiovascular disease and can be used to diagnose many different cardiovascular conditions, including heart failure and valvular disease. Carotid ultrasound is used to screen for atherosclerotic disease in the arteries in the neck, and it was found to improve cardiovascular risk prediction in a study called ARIC.[1] Tests utilizing nuclear imaging, CT scanning, and MRI are highly sensitive and are generally ordered if the results of previous tests require further information about the heart. Nuclear-imaging tests to evaluate blood flow to the heart, or *myocardial perfusion*, are especially helpful in assessing people who have coronary artery disease or who are at risk for developing it. Angiography with CT and MRI, both of which allow physicians to visualize the interior of coronary arteries, are noninvasive alternatives to cardiac catheterization that are often used to rule out heart disease in low-risk individuals. Studies indicate that CT angiography is more accurate at detecting and ruling out coronary artery disease than MRI.[2] CT scanning and MRI are also used at the hospital to evaluate patients with stroke. Finally, coronary artery scans, which incorporate CT, can be ordered for people with chest pain or for individuals at intermediate risk for a heart attack.

Chest X-rays

What it is: A picture of the heart, lungs, and bones of the chest.

Why it is ordered: To show the location and size of the heart and blood vessels, as well as implanted devices such as pacemakers. Changes in the size or shape of your heart can indicate a variety of conditions, including heart failure, congenital heart disease (present at birth), and valvular disease (affecting the heart valves). Chest x-rays can show fluid accumulation around the heart or in the lungs. They can reveal problems with the large blood vessels near the heart, such as aortic aneurysm (swelling of the aorta). They can also detect the presence of *calcium deposits* on heart valves and coronary arteries, which can be a sign of atherosclerotic or other disease.

Where it is done: At a physician's office or in a hospital radiology department.

How long it takes: Approximately five to ten minutes.

You will be asked to stand in front of the x-ray machine and remove all jewelry. Generally two views are taken, one from the back and one from the side. You will need to hold your breath when the x-ray is taken. There is no discomfort, and the level of radiation exposure is very low, comparable to the amount of background radiation a person experiences naturally in the course of daily life over a period of ten days.[3] Let your doctor know if you are pregnant before taking a chest x-ray.

Electrocardiography (ECG or EKG)

What it is: A recording of the heart's electrical activity.

Why it is ordered: To obtain a baseline reading of your heart's electrical activity. Results of this test help your physician diagnose and monitor arrhythmias; heart attack (whether in progress, a part of your medical history, or "silent"—one you were unaware of); increases in size of different parts of the heart; and coronary artery disease. This test is also used to monitor heart function at a routine physical examination.

Where it is done: At a physician's office.

How long it takes: About ten minutes. Actual recording time is three to five minutes.

An ECG machine has three main parts: electrodes, oscilloscope, and recorder. A technician first applies conducting jelly to the electrodes, which are small, self-adhesive pads that detect the heart's electrical impulses, before placing them on your chest, arms, and legs. The oscilloscope is a monitor that shows the heart's electrical impulses. These impulses are translated into written form by the recorder, which produces a tracing on graph paper. Each electrical impulse is recorded as a wave form that is divided into sections P, QRS, and T, which correspond to the different stages in the heart's contraction (see figure 3.2). Grids on the graph paper allow the doctor to measure speed (time) and electrical strength (voltage) of the impulse as it travels through the heart. The ECG can show irregularities in your heart's rhythm or rate, and it can identify damage to the heart muscle from atherosclerotic disease. However, about 50 percent of people with coronary artery disease have completely normal results on electrocardiography.

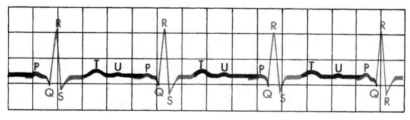

Figure 3.2. The electrocardiogram (ECG) records the electrical activity of the conduction system of the heart. *Illustration by Herbert R. Smith Jr.*

Ambulatory Electrocardiography/Holter® Monitoring

What it is: A continuous monitoring of the heart obtained from a portable ECG machine called a Holter monitor.

Why it is ordered: To evaluate heart rhythm over a longer period of time. This test is also used to monitor the effectiveness of drug therapy for arrhythmias and to assess pacemaker function.

Where it is done: Outside the doctor's office.

How long it takes: Usually twelve to twenty-four hours or longer.

Holter monitoring can detect irregular heart rhythms that occur sporadically outside of the doctor's office, such as following physical exertion. Electrodes are stuck to the chest and connected to a device about the size of a pager, which can be attached to a belt or a shoulder strap. The Holter monitor is battery powered and records information to a cassette tape or, in newer models, to a flash drive. You are expected to continue with normal activities (unless instructed otherwise) with one exception: the equipment must not get wet, so you'll need to temporarily forgo showers and baths. You will be asked to keep a written diary of daily activities, emotional stress, and symptoms so that your doctor can correlate any abnormalities in heart rhythms to your activities at the time. If a longer period of observation is necessary, you may be asked to use a *cardiac event monitor*, which can be worn for weeks or months. There are different kinds of cardiac event monitors. Some record continuously, while others are activated by the patient when he is experiencing symptoms such as dizziness, fainting, palpitations, chest pain, or shortness of breath. They may or may not be attached to the chest with electrodes.

Exercise Stress Testing

What it is: An ECG recording during exercise. Stress tests can also be evaluated using other techniques, such as echocardiography, MRI, and nuclear imaging (see the corresponding sections in this chapter for more information).

Why it is ordered: To diagnose the cause of chest pain and symptoms related to exercise. It may also be used to evaluate the safety of starting a new exercise program or as part of your recovery following a heart attack.

Where it is done: At a doctor's office or exercise lab.

How long it takes: Usually about thirty to sixty minutes.

Exercise stress testing is an extension of ECG. In addition to ECG monitoring with electrodes placed on your chest, arms, and legs, a blood pressure cuff attached to your arm will automatically inflate every few minutes (see figure 3.3). Most stress tests are done while you exercise on a treadmill or ride a stationary bicycle. If you are unable to exercise safely, you may be given a drug intravenously, such as dobutamine, that mimics the effects of exercise on the heart.

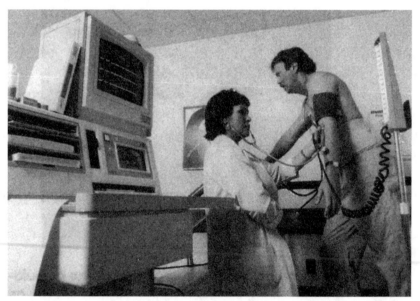

Figure 3.3. During exercise stress testing on a treadmill, blood pressure is monitored *(right)* and an ECG is obtained *(left)*. *Photograph by Herbert R. Smith Jr.*

During the exercise stress test, the intensity of exercise is increased at intervals, which forces the heart to work progressively harder. Exercise is stopped after you reach a predetermined heart rate or develop symptoms. Your heart rate will continue to be monitored for a period of time after exercise. For the test, wear comfortable exercise clothes and athletic shoes. You will be instructed not to eat or drink for three to four hours before the test, especially food and beverages containing caffeine. Ask your doctor whether you should continue taking prescription medications. During the test, tell the technician immediately if you experience symptoms such as chest pain or pressure, shortness of breath, leg pain, dizziness or a feeling of faintness, or mental confusion. Women are more likely to get false-positive results (i.e., the test may indicate they have heart disease when they actually do not), perhaps because they have smaller coronary arteries, which may affect the accuracy of the test.

Echocardiography

What it is: A means of producing a moving picture of the heart and blood vessels by sound waves (ultrasound). It is much more detailed than a chest x-ray and can provide information on the direction and speed of blood flow through arteries.

Why it is ordered: To help doctors diagnose a variety of heart conditions, including impaired heart function, enlargement of the heart, and valvular disease. It can show the size and shape of the heart, its pumping capacity, damage to heart tissues, and abnormalities in the flow of blood through the heart. Echocardiograms can also detect blockages in arteries from atherosclerotic disease. It is often used to determine the *ejection fraction*, which measures how much blood is being pumped out of the heart with each beat.

Where it is done: Usually at a cardiology outpatient diagnostic laboratory.

Echocardiography (sometimes called "echo" for short) is a diagnostic technique that relies on high-frequency inaudible sound waves known as ultrasound. Since it was developed in the 1950s, it has evolved dramatically and can now produce clear, two-dimensional (and even three-dimensional) images. These images often incorporate data obtained from a special type of ultrasound called Doppler ultrasound, which measures the speed of blood traveling through the heart and vessels. Standard ultrasound techniques generally produce two-dimensional, black-and-white images of the heart or vessels, while data from Doppler ultrasound may be presented in colors that refer to patterns of blood flow. Echocardiography is painless and has no known risks or side effects.

Transthoracic Echocardiogram

In a standard echocardiogram, also called a transthoracic echocardiogram, a hand-held device called a *transducer* transmits and receives the ultrasound vibrations. The technician applies gel to enhance sound transmission and presses the tranducer against the chest (see figure 3.4). The sound waves emitted by the transducer cannot be heard or felt. Electrodes will also be attached, so an ECG can be obtained at the same time. You will be asked to lie down, to breathe in and out slowly, and to hold your breath. The "echoes," or reflections, of the sound off the surfaces of the heart are converted into a two-dimensional image that can be displayed on a monitor. The procedure can take up to forty-five minutes. A transesophageal echocardiogram is an alternative, invasive procedure that allows for a clearer view of the heart and is often used to look for blood clots within the chambers of the heart (see the section in this chapter on this procedure).

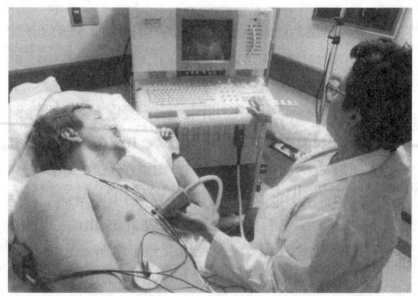

Figure 3.4. A patient undergoing transthoracic echocardiography watches the monitor as the technician holds the transducer against the chest. *Photograph by Herbert R. Smith Jr.*

Stress Echocardiogram

A stress echocardiogram is similar to a conventional exercise stress test (see the previously discussed section on exercise stress testing). Prior to exercise, a standard echocardiogram is obtained. You will then be asked to exercise at increasing levels of intensity, generally on a treadmill, while connected to an ECG. Immediately following exercise, you will lie down, and a repeat echocardiogram will be obtained so that the physician can directly compare the heart's movements before and after exercise. You should allow one and a half to two hours for the entire test. Stress echocardiography can also be performed with drugs that stimulate the heart for people who cannot safely exercise.

Carotid Ultrasound

Ultrasound is widely used to evaluate plaque formation in the carotid arteries of the neck. In particular, it is used to measure the thickness of the artery wall, which is called the carotid intima-media thickness (CIMT), and to determine the speed of blood flow through the artery. CIMT is an indicator of atherosclerosis that may have developed in the carotid arteries. It is related to the likelihood of suffering a future coronary event or stroke and is favorably affected by reducing LDL-C levels. The speed of blood flow through arteries can help doctors locate the site of plaque formation, since velocity increases as the vessel narrows from plaque.

Three-Dimensional Echocardiography

In recent years, faster and more powerful computer processors have paved the way for the development of three-dimensional echocardiography. Although still evolving, this technique allows for the transducer to be held in a fixed position, while a rotating head obtains a series of two-dimensional images that can be reconstructed in three-dimensional form on a video screen or printout. The most advanced transducers can now scan in three dimensions, but the technology for displaying this information has not yet been fully developed. In addition to viewing a three-dimensional image, the doctor can select specific two-dimensional planes for more detailed viewing.

Contrast Echocardiography

Contrast echocardiography is a rapidly evolving field that involves injecting *microbubbles* (extremely small bubbles) intravenously into the circulation. Microbubbles reflect ultrasound waves much more than human tissue, so when they are injected into the bloodstream in low concentrations, they produce greatly enhanced images. A common microbubble contrast agent is a saline (salt) solution that has been shaken vigorously, although there are other commercially developed agents. Contrast echocardiography is safer and less expensive than some of the newer imaging techniques that involve radiation or specialized machines. A disadvantage is that microbubbles do not last very long in the circulation and relatively few make it to the area of interest.

Nuclear Imaging

What it is: Various methods of producing three-dimensional, high-resolution images of the heart's blood flow, structure, and function by injecting a small amount of radioactive particles into the bloodstream.

Why it is ordered: To diagnose coronary artery disease, detect damaged heart tissue, and evaluate the status of the heart muscle.

Where it is done: At a hospital.

Nuclear imaging is a highly specialized field. Generally only hospitals have the extensive resources necessary to maintain the sophisticated machines and radioactive tracers, called *radionuclides*, used in nuclear imaging. Nuclear imaging differs from other imaging techniques because it provides information on how the heart is functioning, as opposed to simply how it looks. It can be combined with computed tomography (CT) and magnetic resonance imaging (MRI) (see the sections in this chapter on CT and MRI). A potential advantage of nuclear imaging compared to standard CT is that it minimizes the amount of exposure to radiation. A small amount of tracer is delivered through an IV needle and is taken up by heart tissues, where it emits radiation that is detected by specialized cameras. The radioactive substance disappears completely from the body within a few days. The amount of radiation exposure varies between one and thirteen times the level of background radiation naturally encountered during the course of one year, depending on the procedure.[4] Repeat tests can increase the cumulative exposure to radiation. Nuclear imaging may also be referred to as *radionuclide imaging, radionuclide angiography, radionuclide ventriculography*, or *nuclear scintigraphy*; these tests show how the different chambers of the heart are functioning, identify damaged tissue, and evaluate blood flow to the heart muscle.

Single Photon Emission Computed Tomography (SPECT)

SPECT is often used to evaluate special stress tests, sometimes called *myocardial perfusion stress tests, nuclear stress tests, multiple gate acquisition (MUGA) scans*, or *thallium heart scans*. SPECT works by injecting a radioactive tracer, such as thallium or technetium, into the bloodstream. The tracer is taken up by tissue in the heart and emits gamma rays, which are detected by a specialized gamma camera that records two-dimensional images. A computer then reconstructs the data into three-dimensional form. These stress tests are used to evaluate myocardial perfusion, or the delivery of nutrients and oxygen to heart tissue, and they can show if there is any tissue that has been damaged by coronary artery disease.

Prior to the test, you may be asked to avoid caffeine, smoking, and food for a period of time. During the test, you will first exercise on a treadmill with an ECG, as in a regular exercise stress test. Then you will receive an IV injection of a radioactive tracer in your arm, and you may be asked to exercise for an additional minute or so, in order for the tracer to be absorbed by the heart muscle. The test can also be conducted by injecting drugs that simulate the effects of exercise on the heart. After lying down on a table for the scan, you need to return about three to four hours later so that another scan can be performed in a resting state (see figure 3.5). The entire test will last about four to five hours. Alternatively, the scan of your heart at rest may be performed before the exercise portion, which may substantially reduce the total time necessary. After the test, you can generally resume normal activities immediately.

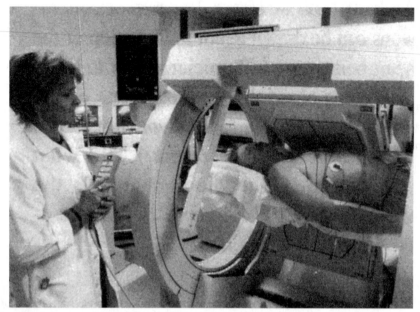

Figure 3.5. A patient undergoing thallium scanning lies still while the equipment is positioned. *Photograph by Herbert R. Smith Jr.*

Positron Emission Tomography (PET)

PET is similar to SPECT, but instead of emitting gamma rays that are measured directly, PET tracers emit positrons. These positrons, which are actually antimatter, then collide with electrons in cells and are annihilated, emitting two gamma photons that are sent out in opposite directions. PET scanners are hollow rings that detect the gamma rays. The data from multiple cross sections is reconstructed to form a three-dimensional image. PET tracers are short-lived and often need to be prepared with an expensive machine called a *cyclotron*, which limits the use of this technology to special cases. PET can be used to evaluate myocardial perfusion, or the delivery of nutrients and oxygen to heart tissue, and to distinguish between heart tissue that is "stunned" (temporarily not working but capable of functioning again) and tissue that has died.

Ultrafast Computed Tomography (CT)

What it is: A technique that uses x-rays to acquire movie-like, three-dimensional views of the beating heart and flowing blood, which can be matched in sequence to the ECG. Electron beam CT (EBCT or EBT) is one form that generates seventeen scans per second. Multidetector CT (MDCT) systems are a newer, faster technology capable of producing even more detailed moving images.

Why it is ordered: To evaluate risk for coronary artery disease by determining if there are calcium deposits or blockages in the coronary arteries.

Where it is done: At a hospital or clinic.

How long it takes: About ten to fifteen minutes.

Ultrafast CT is very useful for generating detailed pictures of the heart and coronary arteries and for conducting coronary calcium scans. *Coronary calcium scans* detect the presence of calcium deposits in the coronary arteries, which can be a sign of atherosclerosis. The results of this test, called the *coronary calcium score*, can help predict your risk of having a future coronary event. Recent studies indicate that the coronary calcium score is good at helping to identify people at moderate risk for a coronary event, although the test is not routinely performed in people without symptoms of heart disease.[5] The routine use of calcium scans has been controversial, in part because of the costs associated with the test. Elderly people may have extensive calcium deposits that are a natural part of aging and may be unrelated to atherosclerosis.

The risk of cancer from radiation exposure is generally low with ultrafast CT, although radiation exposure is higher with MDCT compared to EBCT. Radiation exposure with coronary calcium scoring is comparable to the amount of background radiation a person experiences naturally in the course of daily life over a period of one year.[6] With both MDCT and EBCT machines, you will remove all jewelry and lie down on a sliding table, which will then position you inside a large, hollow tube. Your head will remain outside of the machine, and an ECG will be obtained at the same time. The technician will speak to you through an intercom and may ask you to hold your breath at times. The machine makes clicking and whirring noises as it operates.

CT Angiography

CT angiography is an emerging technology in which a contrast dye is injected into a vein, and an EBCT or MDCT scanner produces a three-dimensional picture of the heart. CT angiography is considered to be a less invasive alternative to standard coronary angiography, which involves the use of a catheter (see the section in this chapter on cardiac catheterization). It is mainly used in patients who come to the hospital with atypical chest pain (probably not related to a heart attack) and who are considered to be at low cardiovascular risk in order to rule out heart disease as the cause of their chest pain. In addition, people who have symptoms and results from exercise stress tests that are suggestive of heart disease, but who are considered to be at low risk for actually having heart disease, may undergo CT angiography in order to avoid invasive angiography. CT angiography can also be used in patients with heart disease to determine the extent of coronary blockages.

During CT angiography, an ECG is obtained at the same time. Injection of the contrast dye may make you feel flushed, warm, or mildly nauseous. The contrast dye contains iodine, and some people may be allergic to it. You may be advised not to eat or drink before the test, and you should drink lots of fluids afterward to flush out the dye. The amount of radiation exposure with the procedure is comparable to the amount of background radiation a person experiences naturally in the course of daily life over a period of five years.[7] The test should take about twenty minutes or up to an hour.

Magnetic Resonance Imaging (MRI)

What it is: A computerized method of scanning that uses radio waves and a powerful magnet.

Why it is ordered: To diagnose coronary heart disease, damage caused by a heart attack, congenital heart disease, cardiomyopathy (enlarged heart), heart failure, pericardial disease (affecting the pericardium, or membrane around the heart), tumors, and valvular disease.

Where it is done: At a hospital or medical imaging facility.

How long it takes: About thirty to sixty minutes.

The MRI scanner is a cylinder about eight feet long with a tunnel running its length. MRI scanners are located in specially built rooms that shield the machine's magnetic field. No metal is allowed inside the room, so you will be asked to fill out a form indicating whether you have a pacemaker, orthopedic pins, or other metal implanted in your body. People with pacemakers cannot have an MRI scan, but other medical devices containing metal are generally safe. All jewelry, coins, and clothing with metal fasteners must be removed. You should also leave credit cards outside because the scanner can damage their magnetic strips. During the test, you will lie on a table that slides into the tunnel. To avoid distorting the images, do not talk or move during the procedure. Expect a noisy experience: the machinery pings and bangs constantly. If you tend to become claustrophobic, tell your doctor in advance, and you may be prescribed a mild sedative. Some newer MRI machines are open on all sides or can be operated while the patient is standing up.

MRI produces cross-sectional images that are generally clearer and more detailed than CT images; it can also generate three-dimensional images. Unlike CT, it does not require exposure to radiation, and it carries no risks. To enhance imaging, you may be injected with a contrast agent, such as gadolinium, that does not contain iodine and may cause a cool sensation. MRI can be used to evaluate stress tests, in which you will be injected with drugs that simulate the effects of exercise on the heart. *Magnetic resonance angiography* (MR angiography or MRA) can also be used to visualize blood vessels throughout the body and detect blockages. It is a noninvasive alternative to standard angiography (see the section in this chapter on angiography), although it is not typically used in routine practice. It is especially recommended for younger patients who may have been born with abnormalities in the coronary arteries. In recent years, high-resolution MRI has been used experimentally to determine whether atherosclerotic plaques are increasing or decreasing in size, and it can be used to evaluate the composition of plaques and the likelihood of plaque rupture.

INVASIVE DIAGNOSTIC PROCEDURES

Sometimes a diagnosis cannot be made with noninvasive tests because the physician needs more information in order to select the best treatment. Some of the procedures considered in this section employ the technique of *cardiac catheterization* in which a long, thin tube is inserted in an artery or vein and guided through the circulation toward the heart. *Angiography*, which is made possible by cardiac catheterization, is a commonly performed invasive diagnostic procedure that produces x-ray images of the heart or blood vessels. Angiographies are usually undertaken when an intervention such as surgery or percutaneous coronary intervention (widening of blocked arteries using special catheters) is being considered (see chapter 5 for more on these procedures). They allow the physician to establish a precise diagnosis, define the extent of disease, make a determination about the need for surgical or medical intervention, and plan the exact procedure to be performed. Sometimes percutaneous coronary intervention may be performed as soon as a blockage is identified during diagnostic testing; at other times, it will be scheduled for a later date. Intravascular ultrasound is generally performed at the same time as other procedures involving cardiac catheterization to provide additional information about atherosclerotic plaques within the arteries. Electrophysiology studies are conducted in people with arrhythmias to identify their source and determine the best course of treatment.

Transesophageal Echocardiography (TEE)

What it is: Similar to a transthoracic echocardiogram (see the previously discussed section on transthoracic echocardiogram) except that a miniature transducer is inserted into the esophagus.

Why it is ordered: To generate clearer images than can be obtained with a transthoracic echocardiogram. To look in the heart chambers for blood clots that can potentially travel through the arteries to other parts of the body.

Where it is done: At a hospital or medical imaging facility.

How long it takes: About ninety minutes.

This is the only diagnostic procedure discussed in this section that does not involve catheterization. Compared to a standard echocardiogram, exceptionally clear images are produced since the transducer is closer to the heart and not blocked by lung tissue. Your doctor will ask you not to eat or drink for four to six hours before the procedure. At the hospital or clinic, the health care team will administer an IV sedative and numb the throat by spraying an anesthetic on it. An ECG will monitor your heart. A technician will place a small, flexible tube called a probe in your throat, and you will be asked to swallow it. As the technician moves the probe into place, you may feel slight discomfort or want to gag, which is normal. Once the probe is in place, you will not feel any pain and may even fall asleep. The probe may be rotated in order to obtain images from different angles. At the end of the test, the probe will be removed, and your heart rate and blood pressure will be monitored as the sedative wears off. You may have a sore throat or difficulty swallowing for a short while after the test.

Cardiac Catheterization

What it is: A technique used to evaluate the heart, including its blood vessels, valves, and muscular wall, by inserting a long, thin tube called a *catheter* into an artery or vein, usually in the arm or groin (see figure 3.6). The catheter is steered to the heart through the circulation using a guide wire, which is removed once the catheter is in place.

Why it is ordered: Cardiac catheterization has many uses: assessing coronary artery disease, including causes of chest pain and complications following heart attack, as well as evaluating congenital heart defects, the heart wall, and valvular disorders. It can be used in an electrophysiologic study to evaluate arrhythmias or with intravascular ultrasound to determine the extent of plaque formation within the arteries (see the final section in this chapter, which discusses intravascular ultrasound). Cardiac catheterization is also the basis for percutaneous coronary interventions (PCI), which are invasive procedures to clear blocked arteries (see chapter 5).

Before the procedure: If you are scheduled for cardiac catheterization, you will not be allowed to have anything to eat or drink for six hours before the procedure. During some procedures, you will be awake so that you can follow instructions from the health care team, or you may be allowed to fall asleep. Either way, physicians and nurses will monitor you continuously throughout the procedure. Expect very little discomfort. About an hour before the procedure starts, you will be given a mild sedative such as diazepam (Valium®) to take by mouth to help you relax. An IV line is inserted to provide fluids and medications. Your doctor will discuss risks and benefits with you before the procedure.

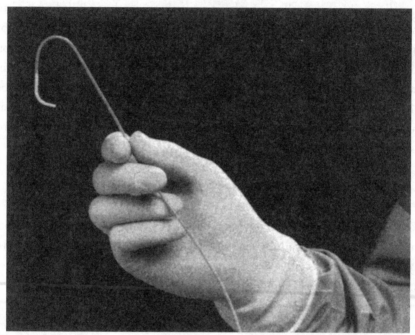

Figure 3.6. A catheter is a long, thin tube that allows doctors to enter and evaluate the cardiovascular system. Specialized catheters can carry tiny instruments and miniature cameras, and they can also be used to administer drugs or contrast solution. *Photograph by Herbert R. Smith Jr.*

During the procedure: Cardiac catheterization is routinely performed on an outpatient basis, often in a cardiac catheterization (cath) lab. The cardiac cath lab is equipped with an x-ray camera called a *fluoroscope*, a video monitor, an ECG unit, and other monitoring equipment. Some rooms are set up with an automated camera that moves around the table; others have a stationary camera, and the table moves from side to side. Cardiac cath labs are also fully equipped in case a cardiac emergency should occur. All the physicians, nurses, and technicians will be wearing surgical gowns, caps, and masks to prevent infection.

ECG electrodes are taped onto the chest, and the area where the catheter will be inserted is shaved and disinfected. Most procedures are now done by puncturing the femoral artery near the groin. Sterile towels, draped around the area, may block your view of what is going on. A local anesthetic is injected, and after the site is numb, a small incision is made in the blood vessel. Expect to feel a slight pressure as the catheter is inserted. Physicians watch the video monitor to guide them in moving the catheter through the body's arteries and positioning it in the heart or coronary arteries. If you feel any chest pain during the procedure, say so.

The procedure takes from half an hour to two hours, depending on how many tests are needed. When the catheter is removed, pressure is applied either by hand or with a special device until blood flow stops. Recently, new devices have been developed that help close the blood vessel and allow you to walk much sooner after the procedure.

After the procedure: Even when cardiac catheterization is done in an out-patient surgery unit, you will be kept in a recovery area and monitored for several hours afterward. The arm or leg with the incision is kept straight and immobile for two to six hours. Nurses check your pulse and blood pressure regularly, and your heartbeat may be monitored by an ECG. Pain medication is available if you need it, and a cold pack may be applied to reduce swelling at the incision area. Before you go home, your physician will discuss the results of your tests with you and let you know whether treatment or more tests will follow. Ask the physician or nurse who is supervising your care any questions you may have.

When you return home: Follow any written instructions the hospital gives you. You may not be allowed to drive home. Unless your doctor says otherwise, you may resume regular activities the next day. The incision area will be sore for several days. Call your doctor if the wound bleeds or if there is any sign of infection—swelling, redness, increased pain, drainage, or fever. There may be a lump, but it will disappear gradually.

Risks are few and rarely serious, with complications occurring in less than

2 percent of patients. Bruising sometimes occurs around the incision, but it disappears. Some of the risks include damage at the site of puncture in the artery, dislodgement of atherosclerotic plaque or blood clots by the catheter, reactions to the contrast dye, and catheter-induced injuries that can very rarely cause an arrhythmia or heart attack.

Angiography

What it is: Angiography, which includes *aortography*, *arteriography*, *coronary angiography*, *pulmonary angiography*, and *ventriculography*, is the x-ray study of the heart and blood vessels during cardiac catheterization. After the catheter is maneuvered into place, contrast solution containing iodine is injected through the catheter into the heart, making it and nearby structures visible with x-rays. Depending on where the catheter is positioned, different areas are studied, including the aorta (the main blood vessel that carries blood from the heart to the rest of the body) and aortic valve (aortography), coronary arteries (arteriography), blood vessels in the lungs (pulmonary angiography), and the lower chambers (ventricles) and valves of the heart (ventriculography).

Why it is ordered: Different types of angiography serve different purposes. Coronary angiography is used to diagnose coronary artery disease by locating the site of atherosclerotic plaques. Aortography can help physicians identify abnormalities of the aorta and assess the aortic valve. Pulmonary angiography may be ordered to evaluate congenital heart disease or pulmonary embolism (blockage in the arteries carrying blood from the heart to the lungs). Ventriculography can detect abnormalities in the contraction of the heart. Other vessels, such as those in the legs or arms or those carrying blood to the brain or specific organs, can also be studied with angiography.

Before the procedure: If you have any allergies or have ever had a reaction to contrast solutions containing iodine, the doctor may order medications to reduce the chance that a reaction will occur during the procedure.

During the procedure: When the contrast solution is first injected, expect to feel a flushing sensation and nausea. Usually this passes within a few seconds. Say something if it does not because the physician can administer a medication to quickly relieve the discomfort. Sometimes people who have not had a previous reaction to iodine will unexpectedly become hypersensitive to it during the test. From time to time, you may be asked to hold your breath, breathe deeply, or cough. Holding your breath during the imaging process ensures better photographic quality, and coughing helps move the contrast solution through the chambers and vessels. Estimates of the radiation exposure associated with angiography using a catheter vary, but are comparable to about one to three years of background radiation exposure typically encountered in everyday life.[8]

After the procedure: You will need to drink plenty of liquids for about eight hours to flush the contrast solution out of your system. You may eat a regular diet unless the doctor orders otherwise.

Electrophysiology Study

What it is: Electrophysiology studies evaluate the heart's electrical conduction system during cardiac catheterization. The catheter helps place electrodes inside the chambers of the heart, where they stimulate different areas of the heart's electrical conduction system. The goal is to pinpoint the exact origin of an irregular heartbeat, or arrhythmia, by re-creating it under controlled circumstances in order to determine the best course of treatment.

Why it is ordered: Electrophysiology studies are ordered when it is necessary to explain an irregular heartbeat, rapid heartbeat, previous cardiac arrest, and fainting.

During the procedure: For electrophysiology studies, the cardiac catheter is usually inserted through the femoral vein in the groin. During the procedure you may feel your heart speed up, slow down, or skip beats. Changes in rhythm during testing are normal; however, report any chest pain or other discomfort you experience. The procedure can take up to six hours or longer. An intervention such as catheter ablation may sometimes be performed at the same time as diagnostic testing (see chapter 6).

After the procedure: You will be asked to remain in bed for two to six hours. A continuous ECG recording will be made during this time.

Intravascular Ultrasound (IVUS)

What it is: A method of obtaining a cross-sectional view of an artery using ultrasound during cardiac catheterization. The tip of the catheter contains a miniature ultrasound probe that emits sound waves from within the blood vessel.

Why it is ordered: IVUS is seldom conducted by itself and is rarely used to make diagnoses. It is usually done at the same time that an invasive procedure, such as percutaneous coronary intervention, is performed, and it provides information about the volume of atherosclerotic plaque within an artery and how much the artery might be blocked. Unlike angiography, IVUS allows plaque to be seen. In recent years, IVUS has been used experimentally to try to determine which plaques are most likely to rupture and cause a heart attack, as well as to document changes in size of atherosclerotic plaques. IVUS is significantly more expensive than angiography.

During the procedure: The catheter is generally inserted through the femoral artery in the groin. The IVUS procedure takes about thirty to sixty minutes.

After the procedure: You will be asked to remain in bed for three to six hours.

***

In the first three chapters of this book, we have discussed how atherosclerosis develops, what you can do to protect yourself from developing atherosclerosis and heart disease, and what tests doctors use to determine whether you might have heart disease. The next two chapters will explain the major forms of atherosclerotic vascular disease and pinpoint available treatment options for these conditions.

CHAPTER 4

ATHEROSCLEROTIC
VASCULAR DISEASE

One of the main functions of blood is to deliver oxygen to tissues and organs throughout the body. The heart itself receives oxygen from blood pumped through the coronary arteries (see figure 4.1). When atherosclerosis develops, the flow of blood and oxygen through an artery is reduced as plaque builds up and clogs the vessel. Doctors refer to a deficiency in the normal supply of blood and oxygen as *ischemia*. Ischemia that affects the heart, also called *ischemic heart disease* or *myocardial ischemia*, can produce a range of conditions, depending on the severity of the blockage(s) in the coronary arteries. Ischemia can sometimes cause permanent damage to organs and tissues. If ischemia is severe enough to cause permanent tissue damage, *infarction* is said to occur, which means that an area of tissue has died. Infarction that occurs in the heart is called a heart attack, or *myocardial infarction*.

In some cases, ischemia and even infarction can be "silent," and the patient may experience no symptoms of heart disease. The American Heart Association (AHA) estimates that 195,000 people each year have a heart attack without noticing any symptoms.[1] Damage from these silent heart attacks is usually detected at a later date on an electrocardiogram (ECG). In other individuals, a blockage of the coronary arteries may not cause symptoms while the person is at rest, but it may be sufficient enough to cause chest pain during periods of physical exertion or stress. Chest pain that occurs only during exercise or stress is called *stable angina*, and it indicates that the heart is not receiving enough oxygen as it is forced to work harder.

143

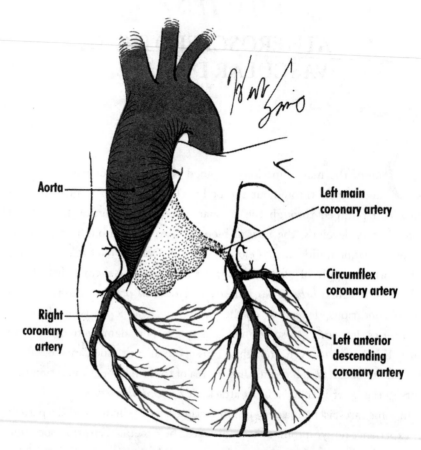

Figure 4.1. The coronary arteries, which arise from the aorta, provide blood to the various tissues of the heart. *Illustration created by Herbert R. Smith Jr.*

Ischemia can become more severe depending on the size and location of the blockage, the stiffness of the blood vessel, and the number of blocked arteries. Atherosclerotic plaques can also rupture, forming a blood clot that then cuts off blood flow. The formation of a blood clot is called thrombosis, and a blood clot is called a *thrombus* (see figure 4.2). The term *vulnerable plaque* refers to plaques that are most prone to rupture. Generally, the plaques that cause heart attacks do not completely block the flow of blood through the artery. Instead, vulnerable plaques may have a lesser degree of blockage, or stenosis, but they are filled with lipid and are more likely to rupture because there is only a thin layer of cells encasing the plaque or because the edges of the plaque have become worn down.

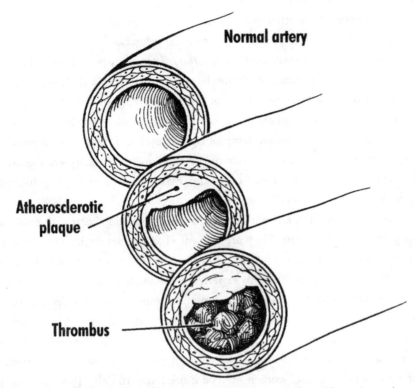

Normal artery

Atherosclerotic plaque

Thrombus

Figure 4.2. Blood flows through the center of a normal artery *(top)*. After atherosclerotic plaque forms, blood flow is restricted *(middle)*. If a blood clot, or thrombus, forms, the artery is blocked *(bottom)*. *Illustration created by Herbert R. Smith Jr.*

Acute coronary syndrome is an umbrella term that refers to chest pain caused by myocardial ischemia that either occurs without physical exertion (at rest) or with progressively less strenuous levels of exertion (the ability to exercise without pain becomes increasingly worse over time). It includes a condition called *unstable angina*, in which chest pain occurs suddenly and sometimes at rest, and two forms of myocardial infarction, or heart attack. During a myocardial infarction, as opposed to unstable angina, cells in the heart die due to lack of oxygen, resulting in irreversible damage to the heart. The two forms of myocardial infarction are differentiated by the extent of the tissue damage they cause, which can often be detected by the results of an ECG. In many cases, an ECG can indicate whether or not blood flow through a coronary artery is likely to have become completely cut off.

Many people have atherosclerosis without experiencing clinical symptoms of heart disease, such as angina or myocardial infarction. Some of these individuals with *subclinical* (asymptomatic) *atherosclerosis* may have undergone tests that identified the presence of atherosclerotic plaques within their arteries, but many will be unaware of the extent of their underlying disease (See chapter 1 for more on the initiation and progression of atherosclerosis). By the time an individual experiences cardiac symptoms, atherosclerosis is often far advanced, frequently affecting more than one of the three major coronary arteries. It is thus essential to control risk factors and maintain a heart-healthy lifestyle *before* symptoms of heart disease appear.

As we discussed in chapter 2, women tend to develop heart disease about ten years later than men. They are also affected differently by heart disease when it does occur, in part because they have smaller hearts and arteries than men. Women are more likely to experience the chest pain of angina as their first symptom of heart disease, whereas men are more likely to suffer a myocardial infarction. Women may experience bouts of angina over a longer period of time before having a heart attack. Perhaps because women are less aware of their risk for heart disease and slower to attribute possible heart attack symptoms to a cardiac cause, women may be more likely to delay in seeking help for a possible heart attack. Yet heart attacks tend to be more severe in women compared to men, so any delay can have negative consequences. Chest pain is the most common symptom of a heart attack in both men and women, but women are more likely to have less common symptoms such as shortness of breath, nausea, fatigue, and jaw pain. By educating themselves, women can be prepared to take action should symptoms of heart disease arise.

This chapter describes the major forms of atherosclerotic vascular disease, with the first three sections focusing on coronary artery disease: stable angina, unstable angina, and myocardial infarction.[2] The fourth section covers peripheral artery disease, which is caused by atherosclerosis of the arteries leading to the legs or arms. The fifth section focuses on atherosclerotic disease of the carotid and cerebral arteries that feed the brain, which can result in an *isch-*

emic stroke or transient ischemic attack (ministroke). All of these forms of atherosclerotic vascular disease are characterized by a reduced flow of blood and oxygen to critical tissues due to stenosis (narrowing of an artery) or by plaque rupture leading to an acute event. Atherosclerosis may also occur in the renal arteries that supply the kidneys, causing renal artery stenosis, and it can contribute to the development of aortic aneurysms (swelling of the aorta), which can rupture suddenly and cause sudden cardiac death.

Each section in this chapter will explain what is happening to the body when an ischemic condition occurs, what course of action you should take if you begin experiencing symptoms, and how each condition will be diagnosed and possibly treated. The particular course of treatment that your doctor ultimately decides upon will depend on many factors, including the severity of atherosclerotic disease and your overall health. This chapter provides a brief summary of which tests or procedures *may* be recommended, depending on your condition. You should refer to chapter 3 for more information on specific diagnostic tests. Chapter 5 contains detailed information on cardiac medications and the procedures commonly used to treat atherosclerotic vascular disease, including percutaneous coronary interventions (PCI) with or without stenting and bypass surgery.

STABLE ANGINA

Characteristics and Causes

Stable angina is chest pain that occurs from myocardial ischemia, primarily after physical exertion. It may also occur in stressful situations, after eating (because blood is diverted to the stomach and intestines), or during cold weather. Stable angina indicates that the heart is generally receiving a constant supply of oxygen, except for when there is an increased demand placed on it. Stable angina is most commonly caused by atherosclerotic plaques that reduce blood flow to the heart. It is also affected by *vasoconstriction*, or the muscular contraction of the walls of an artery. Atherosclerosis can cause arteries to contract abnormally, either by directly damaging the arterial wall or by triggering an increased release of substances that cause arterial narrowing. Cold weather can also cause blood vessels to contract. One trigger of angina is walking uphill in the cold after eating a large meal.

Angina is a common sign of coronary artery disease, although not everyone with coronary artery disease experiences chest pain. The AHA estimates that nine million Americans suffer from stable angina.[3] About 500,000 new cases occur each year. Approximately 18 percent of people with stable angina go on to have a heart attack. Women are more likely to experience the chest pain of angina as their first symptom of heart disease, and they may experience bouts of angina over a longer period of time before having a heart attack.

Stable angina tends to be described more as a feeling of chest discomfort, as opposed to outright pain. The discomfort may feel like a squeezing, crushing, or suffocating pressure against the chest, or it can be a more mild sensation of pressure or heaviness. Some people experience feelings of numbness or burning. Frequently, the discomfort is located directly behind the breastbone, but it also commonly radiates down the inside of the left arm. Some people may experience discomfort down the outsides of both arms or in the back, shoulders, and jaw. After eating, angina can sometimes be mistaken for indigestion, gas pain, or gastroesophageal reflux disease (GERD, acid reflux).

Stable angina usually starts out gradually and lasts for about five minutes or less. It typically disappears after five to fifteen minutes, either after rest or after taking a medication for angina such as nitroglycerin (see chapter 5). Angina that does not disappear after rest or after taking nitroglycerin, or that is not associated with physical exertion, may be unstable angina. Some people with stable angina are only able to exercise a certain amount before experiencing symptoms, while others may have days when they can engage in substantial amounts of physical activity and days when they cannot.

Diagnosis and Management

If you are experiencing chest discomfort following physical activity, you should not ignore it or simply give up exercising. You should consult a doctor for a thorough evaluation and monitoring of your condition. Stable angina is not considered a medical emergency, so by itself does not require calling 9-1-1. If in doubt about whether you might be suffering a heart attack, go immediately to a hospital emergency room. During a regular office visit, the doctor will evaluate your risk factors for heart disease (see chapter 2). Control of cardiovascular risk factors, such as high blood pressure, cigarette smoking, and high cholesterol, is the first step in the treatment of stable angina. Your doctor will likely also recommend lifestyle changes to improve diet and exercise, and possibly medications to control risk factors as well. It is not uncommon for people with stable angina to have high cholesterol levels and other cardiovascular risk factors. As we discussed in previous chapters, it is crucial that people diagnosed with heart disease, including stable angina, achieve LDL-C levels less than 100 mg/dL in order to reduce the risk for future coronary events. If your doctor determines that you are at very high cardiovascular risk, an LDL-C target of less than 70 mg/dL, or even lower, may be appropriate.

Your doctor may conduct exercise stress tests to confirm a diagnosis of coronary artery disease (see chapter 3). ECG results at rest may be normal in people with stable angina. Exercise stress testing using ECG, echocardiography, or thallium-scanning/nuclear-imaging techniques may enable physicians to determine whether you have exercise-induced ischemia. In many cases, stable angina can be treated with medication and lifestyle changes alone. Since several factors can contribute to the imbalance between oxygen supply and demand that characterizes angina, more than one type of medication may be needed. Some of the most common medications used to control angina and protect against future coronary events are nitrates (nitroglycerin), beta-blockers, calcium channel blockers, ACE inhibitors, angiotensin receptor blockers (ARBs), aspirin, and statins (see chapter 5 for information on cardiac medications). Nitrates and calcium channel blockers are *vasodilators*, or agents that relax and dilate blood vessels. Beta-blockers work by decreasing the amount of oxygen needed by the heart and by slowing the heart rate. If symptoms persist with medication or if noninvasive tests indicate that you may have severe blockages in the coronary arteries, invasive testing with coronary angiography (see chapter 3) and procedures such as percutaneous coronary intervention or bypass surgery (see chapter 5) may be recommended.

UNSTABLE ANGINA

Characteristics and Causes

Unstable angina, as the name implies, is not as predictable as angina that occurs due to exercise. You do not have to have had stable angina in order to have unstable angina. Unstable angina is characterized by chest discomfort that occurs at rest or with progressively less intense levels of exertion. It may occur after only minimal exertion, and it typically lasts longer than twenty minutes. Nitroglycerin and rest often fail to relieve the pain. If you have experienced stable angina in the past, signs of unstable angina include attacks that are more severe, longer, or more frequent than before.

Unstable angina may be a sign of an impending heart attack. It is a **medical emergency**, and you should immediately **go to the hospital or call 9-1-1**. Unstable angina is considered an acute coronary syndrome, which means that there is severe myocardial ischemia and your heart is not receiving enough oxygen. Acute coronary syndromes include unstable angina and myocardial infarction. When you arrive at the hospital, health care workers will try to determine whether or not your chest pain is a sign that you are currently experiencing a heart attack. Results of an ECG and of blood tests are used to determine whether your heart tissue has suffered permanent damage (see the section on diagnosis and management of unstable angina). If it has not, then the chest pain is most likely unstable angina and a sign of underlying coronary artery disease.

Unstable angina indicates a greater degree of myocardial ischemia than occurs with stable angina, but less than occurs with a heart attack. With unstable angina, atherosclerotic plaques may have grown large enough to significantly reduce the flow of blood through an artery, or a plaque may have ruptured, forming a blood clot that then partially obstructs an artery. In both cases, the supply of oxygen to the heart is significantly diminished, resulting in severe chest pain. In addition, vasoconstriction (muscular contraction of arteries) as a result of atherosclerosis may play a role in unstable angina.

Variant (Prinzmetal's) Angina

Variant or Prinzmetal's angina is a rare type of angina. It can occur in patients with or without coronary atherosclerosis. In variant angina, a sudden spasm causes a coronary artery to contract severely, resulting in a sharp, dramatic reduction in the supply of oxygen to the heart. This type of spasm is different from typical vasoconstriction. It is much more intense and occurs at one point in the artery, rather than throughout a larger segment. Symptoms of variant angina generally occur at rest and are not associated with exercise or emotional stress. The pain is severe and may be accompanied by fainting. Attacks often happen between midnight and eight o'clock in the morning and sometimes occur in clusters of two or three within a time span of thirty to sixty minutes. People with variant angina tend to be younger than people with stable or unstable angina, and many are heavy cigarette smokers. Variant angina produces a specific abnormal pattern on the ECG, which is typically how the condition is diagnosed. Nitroglycerin generally brings relief from symptoms. Patients may also be prescribed calcium channel blockers, but beta-blockers and aspirin may actually worsen the condition in some patients (see chapter 5). Stopping smoking is strongly advised for all individuals, but particularly for individuals with this condition.

Diagnosis and Management

Upon arriving at the hospital with acute chest pain, one of the first things the hospital staff will try to determine is if you are currently undergoing a heart attack. You may be evaluated in a "chest pain unit" before being admitted to the hospital. Two of the first tests you will be given are an ECG and a blood test. These tests will likely also be repeated throughout your hospital stay in order to monitor any changes that may occur. On an ECG, the heartbeat is divided into sections P, QRS, and T, which correspond to the different stages in the heart's contraction (see figure 3.2 in chapter 3). The ST-segment of the ECG provides information regarding myocardial ischemia. In the most serious form of a heart attack, the ST-segment is elevated, which indicates that part of the heart tissue is not receiving any blood flow and that a coronary artery is most likely completely blocked by plaque or a blood clot. This type of heart attack is termed an *ST-elevation myocardial infarction* (STEMI), and blood flow through the heart needs to be restored as quickly as possible.

If the ST-segment is depressed, there may be severe ischemia, and the coronary arteries are most likely only partially blocked. Sometimes the ST-segment will not be elevated, but there may be changes in it that suggest a high risk for complications or another coronary event. In both cases, the type of heart attack is called a *non-ST-elevation myocardial infarction* (NSTEMI). Both NSTEMI and unstable angina are serious conditions that a physician can decide to treat either aggressively, by going ahead with an invasive intervention as soon as possible, or conservatively, by treating with medications first and considering invasive strategies later. These two acute coronary syndromes can be distinguished by the results of a blood test that indicates whether heart tissue has died. In patients with unstable angina, levels of cardiac enzymes are often normal, whereas with NSTEMI, they are elevated, indicating cellular death. The cardiac enzymes measured are troponin T or I and creatine kinase (CK-MB), which are released when heart tissue dies. Depending on the results of the ECG and the blood test, a stress test will sometimes be performed in the hospital, at discharge, or at a later date.

Patients with unstable angina are generally admitted to the hospital, possibly to a coronary care unit, and monitored continuously with an ECG while resting in bed. Supplemental oxygen may be provided. Unless patients are intolerant of aspirin, aspirin tablets to prevent blood clotting are given as soon as possible and continued indefinitely. Other drugs to prevent clotting (*antithrombotic drugs*) will also be administered intravenously or orally. Drugs to reduce chest pain and decrease the demand for oxygen by the heart, called *anti-ischemic drugs*, may be administered intravenously or orally. If chest pain persists, patients may be given morphine. If necessary, they may be given medications to improve the function of the *left ventricle*, which is the chamber of the heart responsible for pumping blood to the rest of the body. Lipid-lowering therapy with statins may also be prescribed or administered. In addition to lowering cholesterol levels, statins protect against future coronary events when given immediately following an acute coronary syndrome. Major clinical trials have shown that high doses of statins can reduce the risk for death, a recurrent coronary event, and invasive procedures if given within forty-eight hours of an acute coronary syndrome.[4]

After the patient with unstable angina receives a variety of medications, the doctor and patient have a choice between an early invasive strategy or a more conservative approach. With the early invasive strategy, a doctor goes ahead with cardiac catheterization as soon as possible, generally within four to twenty-four hours of hospital admission, in order to determine the extent of coronary blockage using angiography (see chapter 3). If feasible, angiography is followed immediately by *revascularization* (restoration of blood flow) with percutaneous coronary intervention (PCI) or, if necessary, through bypass surgery (see chapter 5). With a more conservative approach, a doctor waits to see whether drug therapy is sufficient to prevent further chest pain and will schedule a noninvasive stress test. Invasive tests and procedures are then considered as appropriate in the future. Sometimes the choice of treatment depends on the available hospital facilities, as smaller hospitals may not always have a cardiac cath lab.

If you are admitted to the hospital with unstable angina and do not undergo invasive procedures, you will probably be monitored for at least twenty-four hours. When you are discharged, your doctor will likely stress the importance of controlling cardiovascular risk factors to prevent future coronary events (see chapter 2). You may be prescribed lipid-lowering statins, beta-blockers, medications to control high blood pressure, ACE inhibitors or ARBs, or aspirin or another anticlotting drug, if you are not already taking them.

MYOCARDIAL INFARCTION

Characteristics and Causes

Most heart attacks are caused when an atherosclerotic plaque ruptures, allowing clotting substances from the blood into the artery wall: platelets in the blood will cluster in response, and a clot forms to block the artery, either partially or entirely. In addition, atherosclerosis makes arteries stiff and prone to vasoconstriction, which further diminishes blood flow. During a heart attack, or myocardial infarction, the obstruction of blood flow to the heart is so severe that tissue begins to die.

This is why prompt action when a heart attack hits is so important.

Any delay may increase chances of heart damage and hurt chances of survival. Unfortunately, some people who have heart attacks soon develop a fatal heart rhythm called ventricular fibrillation and die suddenly after the onset of symptoms (see chapter 6 for more on arrhythmias). However, the AHA estimates that almost two-thirds of people who suffer an acute myocardial infarction survive the immediate event. Of those who die, about half do so before reaching a hospital. A suspected heart attack is a **medical emergency** that requires immediate transport to the hospital. Time is of the essence in order to prevent further tissue death and the development of abnormal heart rhythms.

More than 60 percent of heart attack victims experience classic indicators of heart difficulty days to weeks before the heart attack occurs (see figure 4.3). They may have unstable angina that is accompanied by shortness of breath and a pervasive feeling of being extremely tired. Classic warning signals of a heart attack experienced by men and women include pain, sweating, nausea, sensations of indigestion or burning, and feelings of faintness. Ways to identify a heart attack are the frequency of the chest pain, its duration and intensity, and its failure to be relieved by rest or nitroglycerin. The pain is generally severe and sometimes intolerable, and it can last for more than thirty minutes to a few hours. Men may be more likely to report that the pain gets better with rest.

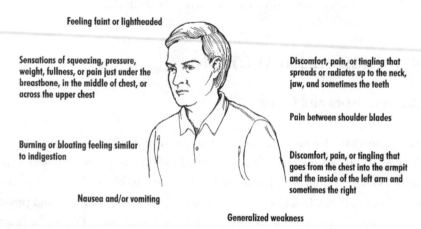

Feeling faint or lightheaded

Sensations of squeezing, pressure, weight, fullness, or pain just under the breastbone, in the middle of chest, or across the upper chest

Discomfort, pain, or tingling that spreads or radiates up to the neck, jaw, and sometimes the teeth

Pain between shoulder blades

Burning or bloating feeling similar to indigestion

Discomfort, pain, or tingling that goes from the chest into the armpit and the inside of the left arm and sometimes the right

Nausea and/or vomiting

Generalized weakness

Figure 4.3. Classic warning signals of a heart attack. *Illustration created by Herbert R. Smith Jr.*

Women may be more likely than men to describe atypical chest pain, such as a feeling of tightness in the chest that comes and goes. Weakness, lethargy, breathlessness, or nausea may be the key symptom in women, and there may be a sensation of inhaling cold air. Often, women are slower to attribute these signals to a heart attack and are more likely to postpone seeking help during this critical period. Their symptoms may also be less severe. As a result, they are more likely to have undiagnosed heart disease and to be undertreated by physicians.

Sometimes cocaine use can cause severe chest pain, ECG changes, and myocardial ischemia in people who do not have evidence of coronary atherosclerosis. The effects of cocaine increase the demand for oxygen by the heart, constrict blood vessels, and can make blood more likely to clot. In some people, cocaine use can trigger a heart attack, while in others it can cause symptoms that mimic a heart attack. The risk is highest one hour after ingestion and then rapidly declines. Sometimes cocaine-related chest pain is not directly related to the heart at all and may instead be due to a painful irritation of the membrane surrounding the lungs.

Responding to a Heart Attack

Chest pain that lasts longer than twenty minutes suggests a heart attack or unstable angina and demands immediate transport to a hospital. If you experience pain in the center of the chest that radiates to the shoulders, neck, or arms and you feel faint or nauseated, or you experience shortness of breath or sudden sweating, **go immediately to a hospital or call 9-1-1**. Do not worry about feeling embarrassed if you go to an emergency room unnecessarily.

Knowing where to go if you or someone you know has a heart attack can save time. Plan in advance. Contact the hospitals near your home and office to identify those that provide twenty-four-hour emergency cardiac care. If you have heart disease, you should locate the nearest facility that has a cardiac cath lab and is capable of performing percutaneous coronary intervention (PCI) or bypass surgery. Some ambulances, particularly in large cities, are equipped to perform tests and administer medications that will expedite treatment once the vehicle arrives at the hospital. If you need to call an ambulance to take you to the hospital, call 9-1-1 first and call your doctor second. Don't delay by first trying to reach your doctor for advice. Every minute counts.

Diagnosis and Management

Upon arriving at the hospital, the results of a blood test and ECG will help doctors confirm if you are experiencing a heart attack and, if so, how best to treat it. An ECG may be obtained in the ambulance if available; repeat or continuous ECG monitoring at the hospital is likely. Elevated levels of the cardiac enzymes troponin T or I and creatine kinase (CK-MB) indicate that heart tissue is dying and that you are suffering a myocardial infarction. An elevation of the ST-segment on an ECG indicates that a coronary artery is most likely completely blocked by plaque or a blood clot. This type of heart attack is called an ST-elevation myocardial infarction (STEMI). If the ST-segment is not elevated, then there is severe ischemia, but the coronary arteries are most likely only partially blocked. This type of heart attack is called a non-ST-elevation myocardial infarction (NSTEMI).

Patients with STEMI require immediate revascularization, or restoration of blood flow to the heart. Revascularization for STEMI patients can be achieved with drugs to break up blood clots, called *thrombolytic* or *fibrinolytic therapy*; with an invasive procedure to unblock clogged arteries; or with both. The factors that affect the decision between thrombolytic therapy and an invasive procedure, as well as the factors that affect which type of invasive procedure is performed (percutaneous coronary intervention versus bypass surgery), are discussed further in chapter 5.

Patients with NSTEMI may be treated either aggressively, by going ahead with an invasive intervention (percutaneous coronary intervention or bypass surgery) as soon as possible, or conservatively, by treating with cardiac medications first and considering invasive strategies depending on the results of noninvasive tests. Invasive management is the preferred strategy for more at-risk patients.

Patients with both types of heart attack will receive a number of cardiac medications while at the hospital. Aspirin tablets will be given as soon as possible and continued indefinitely in order to prevent further blood clotting. Other intravenous and oral medications to prevent the formation of new blood clots, such as clopidogrel or intravenous heparin, are also administered. Drugs to address chest pain will be given because pain stimulates the nervous system, which is already being taxed because of the heart attack itself. Patients may receive a variety of drugs to reduce the load placed on the heart and to increase blood flow to the heart, such as nitrates, beta-blockers, and calcium channel blockers. Other medications may be administered depending on the specific damage done to the heart or if there are complications following the heart attack.

Unless there are complications, patients undergoing bypass surgery generally remain in the hospital for four to seven days. After percutaneous coronary intervention, patients often leave the hospital the following day. Upon discharge, you will likely receive counseling about the importance of lifestyle modifications to control cardiovascular risk factors (see chapter 2). You may also be prescribed a variety of medications, including lipid-lowering statins, blood pressure medication, nitrates, beta-blockers, ACE inhibitors, ARBs, and anticlotting agents, if you are not already taking them.

The Heart after a Myocardial Infarction

After a heart attack, the tissue that has died is eventually replaced by scar tissue, a process that usually takes about one month. In some individuals, a myocardial infarction may stimulate the development of *collateral circulation*. If an artery is blocked, sometimes a system of small vessels will develop to provide a detour around the blockage (see figure 4.4). Collateral circulation may help people with heart disease to a certain extent by providing alternate routes of blood flow to the heart. Everyone has collateral vessels at birth, but they do not always become functional. Some people are unable to develop collateral circulation. In others, exercise may aid in the development of collateral circulation.

The damage incurred to the heart during a heart attack can sometimes lead to the chronic chest pain of angina or to other long-term complications. Arrhythmias, or abnormal heart rhythms, and heart failure, in which the heart's pumping capacity is insufficient to meet the body's demands, are two common complications. More than 90 percent of heart attack survivors develop arrhythmias, often within the first twenty-four hours following a heart attack. The risk for heart failure is increased if the left ventricle (the lower chamber of the heart responsible for pumping blood out to the rest of the body) is damaged (*left ventricular dysfunction*). About 30 percent of people who experience a heart attack progress to heart failure. In many cases, arrhythmias and heart failure can be managed with medications. Chapters 6 and 7 discuss the various forms of arrhythmia and heart failure, as well as the different treatment options for these conditions.

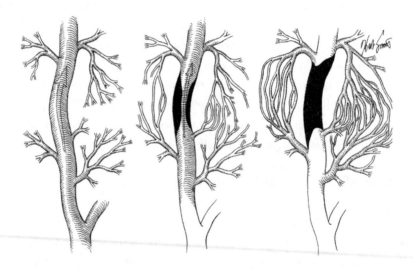

Figure 4.4. Nature can compensate for vessels blocked by atherosclerotic disease with collateral circulation, a network of small arteries and capillaries that detour around the obstruction. *Illustration created by Herbert R. Smith Jr.*

As discussed in chapter 2, once someone has suffered a heart attack, the chances of experiencing another heart attack or a stroke greatly increase. For this reason, it is very important to take control by optimizing your cardiovascular risk factors. Pay careful attention to the advice your doctor gives you, make sure to take all prescribed medications and, under supervision, gradually begin to implement a program of healthy eating and exercise. Also, see chapter 5 for information on cardiac rehabilitation.

PERIPHERAL ARTERY DISEASE

Characteristics and Causes

Peripheral artery disease (PAD) most commonly affects the legs and results when atherosclerosis develops in the arteries that provide blood to the peripheral tissues (such as the limbs). Many people with PAD also have coronary artery disease. Atherosclerotic plaques that block the flow of blood to the legs generally develop in one of two places (see figure 4.5). In the first pattern of disease, the abdominal aorta, which is the major artery in the abdomen, or the iliac arteries in the pelvis become blocked, cutting off blood flow. This condition may be referred to as *aortoiliac disease* or as *Leriche's syndrome* after the French surgeon who originally described it. In the second pattern of disease, the femoral arteries in the thighs become blocked. Some people may have plaques in both of these locations. Blockage may also occur in the arteries below the knees and in the arms. As with coronary artery disease, arteries affected by atherosclerosis tend to be stiff and more prone to constriction, which further decreases blood flow through the vessels.

Approximately eight million individuals in the United States are estimated to have PAD.[5] Risk factors for cardiovascular disease—including high cholesterol and high blood pressure—also contribute to the development of PAD (see chapter 2 for information on risk factors). Cigarette smoking and diabetes confer especially increased risk for PAD. Approximately 90 percent of people with symptoms of PAD are current or former smokers. Continuing to smoke with PAD increases the chances of critical limb ischemia and limb loss.

The primary symptom of PAD is *intermittent claudication*, which is a pain, ache, sense of fatigue, or discomfort that occurs with exercise such as walking and that disappears with rest. As with stable angina, intermittent claudication indicates that the affected muscles are not receiving enough oxygen as physical activity increases. In most patients, symptoms develop gradually over time. In patients with the aortoiliac pattern of disease, pain typically occurs in the buttocks, hips, or thighs. Calf pain is a common complaint and occurs when the lower arteries in the leg are affected. Pain may also be felt in the ankles, feet, shoulders, biceps, or forearms, depending on the location of

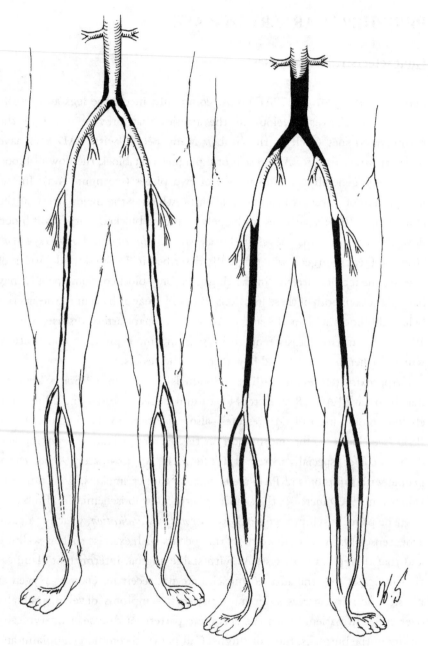

Figure 4.5. Typical patterns of atherosclerotic disease in the abdominal aorta and vessels to the legs. Usually there is a gradual progression from mild to moderate blockage *(left)* to complete obstruction *(right)*. *Illustration created by Herbert R. Smith Jr.*

stenosis (narrowing of arteries). Symptoms may be triggered by walking at a certain speed, for a particular distance, or up an incline, and they typically resolve after several minutes of rest. People with PAD cannot walk as fast or for as long as people without PAD. Cramps in the calves or thighs that occur at night, commonly called "charley horses," may sometimes be confused for intermittent claudication but are not a symptom of PAD. Having "restless legs" at night is not associated with PAD.

As PAD worsens, claudication becomes more severe, and the ability to walk becomes more limited. Eventually pain may be felt even at rest. Pain at rest is called *critical limb ischemia* and is characterized by atrophy (shrinking or wasting away) of the muscles and fat in the legs, coldness of the feet, loss of hair, paleness or blueness in the legs, and thickened and brittle toenails. The skin of the legs may be very sensitive to pain, and eventually leg ulcers and gangrene may begin to develop.

Diagnosis and Management

A diagnosis of PAD can generally be made based on the symptoms described above. In addition, doctors can often determine which artery is blocked by observing the limbs and checking the pulses at different parts of the legs. A bruit may be heard over a partially obstructed artery, and the pulse in the leg or foot below the blockage may be faint or absent. The *ankle/brachial index* (ABI) is an easily obtained measurement that is often used to confirm a diagnosis of PAD. Normally, the blood pressure at the ankle is greater than in the brachial artery of the arm. In healthy individuals, the ratio of the blood pressure at the ankle to the blood pressure in the arm, or the ankle/brachial index, should be 1.0 or greater. Progressive narrowing of the arteries in the legs due to atherosclerosis reduces blood pressure to the ankle, which decreases the ankle/brachial index. For this test, blood pressure measurements may be obtained using a handheld Doppler ultrasound probe. Patients with intermittent claudication generally have ABI values between 0.5 and 0.8, whereas those with severe leg ischemia may have values below 0.5.

Exercise stress testing with measurements of the ABI at rest and after exercise may be performed in order to evaluate the patient's walking capacity.

This test may also include monitoring of the heart with an electrocardiogram. Noninvasive imaging tests using echocardiography, magnetic resonance angiography, and computed tomography angiography can provide visualization of the peripheral arteries and the extent of plaque blockage. Coronary angiography may be conducted prior to an invasive revascularization procedure in the peripheral tissues since patients with PAD often also have coronary atherosclerosis and experience a high rate of coronary events (see chapter 3 for information on diagnostic testing).

One goal of treatment for PAD is to prevent a future cardiovascular event, so lifestyle modifications and control of cardiovascular risk factors, including high cholesterol, cigarette smoking, and high blood pressure, are crucial. In evaluating a patient's cardiovascular risk, PAD is considered a "coronary risk equivalent," since many people with PAD go on to have a coronary event. Thus, individuals with PAD should have an LDL-C level less than 100 mg/dL, and preferably less than 70 mg/dL or even lower (see chapter 2 for more on risk factors). Antiplatelet drugs to prevent blood clotting may be prescribed in order to reduce the chances of suffering a heart attack or stroke. Another goal of treatment is to decrease symptoms of intermittent claudication. Currently, two drugs are approved in the United States for this purpose: cilostazol and pentoxifylline (see chapter 5). Supervised exercise training programs have also been shown to reduce symptoms of PAD and improve exercise capacity.

For patients with critical limb ischemia, revascularization with thrombolytic (clot-busting) drugs, percutaneous intervention with or without stenting of the blocked vessel, or bypass surgery is necessary to restore blood flow and prevent loss of limb (see chapter 5 for information on drug and surgical treatments). These procedures may also be considered in patients with intermittent claudication if symptoms do not improve with drug therapy.

ISCHEMIC STROKE AND TRANSIENT ISCHEMIC ATTACK (TIA)

Characteristics and Causes

A stroke, or *cerebrovascular accident* (CVA), results when disruption of the normal blood flow to a portion of the brain causes damage to brain tissue. About 15 to 20 percent of strokes are caused by hemorrhage, in which a cerebral artery bursts and blood flows into the brain or between the brain and the skull. Hemorrhagic stroke is not generally associated with atherosclerosis. About 80 to 85 percent of strokes are ischemic strokes. Ischemic strokes can occur when normal blood flow to the brain is blocked, usually by a blood clot (see figure 4.6). A blood clot can form when an atherosclerotic plaque ruptures in the cerebral arteries in the brain or in the carotid or vertebral arteries in the neck. A clot may also form in the heart or another part of the body and travel in the bloodstream to block a cerebral artery in the brain. This kind of traveling blood clot is called an *embolus* (as opposed to a thrombus, which does not move). If blood flow stops completely for as little as four minutes, the nerve cells in the brain, called *neurons*, begin to die. Neurons can survive reduced blood flow if full flow is reestablished within a few hours.

Risk factors for cardiovascular disease, including age, high blood pressure, diabetes, elevated cholesterol levels, and smoking, also increase the risk for ischemic stroke. High blood pressure is the most common treatable risk factor for stroke, and it has the strongest direct relationship to increased risk. It increases stroke risk by four to six times. Heart disease also increases the risk of stroke, particularly in people who have suffered a recent heart attack or who have heart failure. Risk for a recurrent stroke is high in individuals who have already experienced a stroke or a TIA.

The symptoms of stroke occur suddenly and depend on the area of the brain affected. The single most common symptom is headache. Paralysis, or a weakness or loss of function in an arm, a leg, or a region of the body, such as the face, is a typical sign of stroke. Speech is commonly affected, due to weakness of the tongue on one side of the mouth, causing slurring of speech. At times, the ability to understand language or produce words is impaired.

Less commonly, sensation on one side of the body is affected, and the patient complains of numbness. Vision can be affected in a variety of ways, including loss of vision in one eye, blurring or partial loss of vision (such as to either the left or right side) in both eyes, double vision, or difficulty in focusing. Loss of coordination or loss of balance may result, as can confusion or dizziness. Strokes can occur at any time. The sudden onset of any of the above symptoms is a **medical emergency**, and you should immediately **call 9-1-1**.

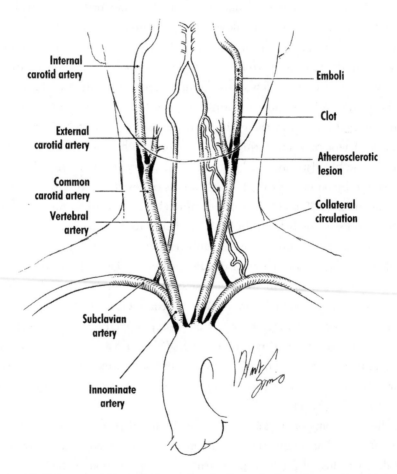

Figure 4.6. Common patterns of atherosclerotic disease in the major arteries supplying blood to the brain. A clot may form at one of these sites, and pieces may break off to form an embolus, which can pass through the blood stream to block vessels in the brain and cause a stroke. *Illustration created by Herbert R. Smith Jr.*

A transient ischemic attack occurs when a clot temporarily blocks the flow of blood and oxygen to the brain. The patient experiences the symptoms of a stroke, but only for a short period of time, typically less than five minutes. With TIA, as opposed to a stroke, symptoms are completely reversible within twenty-four hours (they cause no permanent damage). The brief nature of the symptoms leads many individuals to wait before seeking medical attention. However, if you experience symptoms of a stroke, even briefly, you should go to a hospital emergency room, because you cannot distinguish a stroke from a TIA as it is occurring based on symptoms alone. Although TIAs do not cause permanent brain injury, more than one-third of people who have had a TIA go on to have a stroke. If your doctor determines that you have suffered a TIA, you will likely need to begin treatment to prevent a future stroke from occurring.

Diagnosis and Management

When symptoms of a stroke develop, you should seek emergency medical attention. At the hospital, a CT scan of the brain is usually done first to determine whether you are suffering an ischemic stroke, as opposed to a hemorrhagic stroke or other condition. If an ischemic stroke is identified, drugs to break up blood clots (thrombolytic therapy) and prevent additional clots from forming are immediately administered. Thrombolytic therapy needs to be administered within three hours (at some hospitals, within four and a half hours) following the start of symptoms, so don't delay in calling 9-1-1 if you begin experiencing symptoms of a stroke.

An MRI scan may also be performed to detect ischemic injury to the brain. If it appears that the stroke is a result of a blood clot, tests will be performed to determine whether arteries, especially the carotid arteries in the neck, are narrowed or blocked due to atherosclerotic plaque build-up. These imaging tests may include carotid ultrasound, magnetic resonance angiography, computed tomography angiography, or standard angiography of the cerebral artery in the brain (see chapter 3 for more on diagnostic tests). Electrocardiography may be employed to determine whether abnormal heart rhythms may be contributing to the formation of blood clots. Echocardiography, usually transesophageal echocardiography, may be used to evaluate the heart's pumping action or to search for blood clots within the heart. Patients with TIAs may undergo similar tests in order to determine the underlying cause.

Patients with significant narrowing in the carotid arteries may be considered for surgical removal of the blockage. People who have suffered a stroke or a TIA and who have 60 percent or more blockage may undergo carotid endarterectomy, a surgical procedure to remove plaque in the carotid arteries (see chapter 5). A percutaneous intervention in the carotid arteries with stenting is a newer treatment option. Long-term prevention of stroke includes anticlotting medication and treatment of risk factors for stroke, such as hypertension. Lipid lowering with statins has also been shown to decrease the risk of a recurrent ischemic stroke or TIA.

•••

The next chapter describes options for the medical and surgical treatment of the major forms of atherosclerotic disease discussed in this chapter.

CHAPTER 5
TREATING ATHEROSCLEROTIC
DISEASE IN THE 21st CENTURY

Risk factor modification is the key to preventing the development of atherosclerotic disease. Medication and invasive procedures, including *percutaneous interventions* and surgery, are the remedies once atherosclerotic disease has already developed. As we mentioned earlier, improvements in risk factor control, as well as better medications and hospital interventions, have resulted in a decline in deaths from cardiovascular disease over the past three decades. In the twenty-first century, our ability to treat atherosclerotic disease, relieve symptoms, and improve survival and quality of life is greater than ever before. If you have developed coronary artery disease, peripheral artery disease, or atherosclerotic disease in the carotid or cerebral arteries, this chapter describes the various drugs that may be administered and the procedures that may be performed to treat your condition.[1] It is important to note that these interventions, although often very effective, do not provide a "cure" for atherosclerotic disease. Atherosclerosis will continue to develop unless you make a concerted effort to control your risk factors by eating better, exercising more, losing weight, and stopping smoking.

MEDICAL THERAPY

Many of the drugs discussed in this chapter are also used to treat other heart conditions. For example, beta-blockers, which are used to relieve the chest pain of angina, are also used to control high blood pressure and to treat arrhythmias and heart failure, in addition to other noncardiac conditions. This chapter focuses on the drug effects that are particularly useful for the treatment of atherosclerotic disease. In general, the medications considered in this section combat the effects of reduced blood flow to the heart (anti-ischemic drugs), protect against recurrent cardiovascular events and heart failure (angiotensin-converting enzyme, or ACE, inhibitors and angiotensin receptor blockers, or ARBs), prevent blood clotting (antiplatelet and anticoagulant drugs), and dissolve blood clots (thrombolytic drugs).

Anti-ischemic Drugs

Anti-ischemic drugs have two primary effects: 1) they reduce the demand for oxygen by the heart, and 2) they increase blood flow to the heart. The various classes of anti-ischemic drugs work in different ways to achieve these effects. For example, they can reduce heart rate and blood pressure, they can make the heart contract less forcefully, and they can widen blood vessels. Anti-ischemic drugs are sometimes used to treat the chest pain associated with stable angina and in the hospital during acute coronary syndromes.

Nitrates

Nitrates, which include nitroglycerin, are among the oldest cardiac medications. They remain an important therapy for angina today. Nitrates are vasodilators, or agents that widen blood vessels. Although they have effects on both arteries and veins, their primary effect is to dilate veins, which reduces the heart's workload by making it easier for blood to circulate. The most common side effect is headache. Low blood pressure can be a problem in elderly individuals. Nitrates can cause a serious, potentially fatal drop in blood pressure in men who have taken sildenafil (Viagra®); be sure to tell your doctor if you use this medication.

Nitrates are available in several forms: nitroglycerin tablets, long-acting oral medications, nitroglycerin ointment, nitroglycerin patches, nitroglycerin spray, and intravenous nitroglycerin. Nitroglycerin in all formulations can lose its effectiveness when used repeatedly; this is called nitrate tolerance. As a result, your doctor may schedule your dosages to accommodate a twelve-hour "off" period each day. Nitroglycerin tablets placed under the tongue are the most common formulation. The medication goes to work within five minutes. Nitroglycerin tablets tend to lose their potency, especially when exposed to light, so they should be stored in their original containers. Long-acting oral agents, including isosorbide dinitrate, isosorbide 5-mononitrate, and sustained-release nitroglycerin tablets, are prescribed to be taken between one and three times per day. The nitroglycerin ointment is applied to paper strips between one-half to two inches long and then stuck to the skin, generally in the chest area. It is typically applied every four to six hours and begins working in about thirty minutes. Nitroglycerin patches, which adhere to the skin, can deliver sustained-release nitroglycerin. They typically remain on the skin for as long as twelve hours per day but are removed for twelve hours at night to prevent the development of tolerance. The nitroglycerin spray is used to place droplets onto or under the tongue and should not be inhaled. It can be used five to ten minutes before activities that may cause angina, such as exercise. Intravenous nitroglycerin is used in the hospital to reduce chest pain in individuals suffering acute coronary syndromes.

Beta-Blockers

Beta-blockers are used to treat stable angina, to decrease the load on the heart and reduce chest pain during acute coronary syndromes, and as part of long-term therapy following a heart attack. Beta-blockers work by decreasing the amount of oxygen needed by the heart. They slow the heart rate, decrease blood pressure, and lessen the muscular contractions of the heart at rest and during exercise. During times of stress or exercise, they block the nerve impulses that stimulate the heart. They can help decrease the frequency and severity of angina attacks, and they improve exercise tolerance. Beta-blockers used for the treatment of stable angina include atenolol (Tenormin®), metoprolol (Lopressor®, Toprol-XL®), nadolol (Corgard®), and propranolol (Inderal®).

When given in the hospital to patients with acute coronary syndromes, beta-blockers may be administered intravenously first, followed by oral tablets for the long term. Following a heart attack, beta-blockers have been shown to significantly increase survival and may be prescribed indefinitely. Specific drugs for this purpose include atenolol, metoprolol, and propranolol.

Beta-blockers are classified as cardioselective or noncardioselective. *Cardioselective drugs* work primarily on receptors in the heart muscle. *Noncardioselective drugs* affect receptors in the heart, as well as receptors located in blood vessels and airways. Their differing side-effect profiles may determine which type of drug will work best for you. Breathing difficulties and a worsening of circulatory problems are two of the most serious potential side effects. Since cardioselective drugs target the heart more precisely, they do not affect the airways and blood vessels as much as noncardioselective drugs. At lower dosages, cardioselective drugs are thus less likely to aggravate asthma, bronchitis, or poor circulation in the legs and feet. At higher dosages, however, cardioselective drugs become less "selective" and may cause these kinds of side effects as well.

Beta-blockers in general have a wide range of other potential side effects, including a slow resting heart rate, cold hands and feet, erectile dysfunction, mental and physical slowness and fatigue, depression, nightmares, memory problems, gastrointestinal upset, and low blood sugar in diabetics (as well as a decreased ability to recognize the signs of low blood sugar). Some side effects will diminish with time, but if you find that persistent side effects are affecting your quality of life, you may want to ask your doctor about switching to a different beta-blocker or adjusting dosages.

Calcium Channel Blockers

Calcium channel blockers (CCBs) are vasodilators (agents that cause blood vessels to relax and widen) that work by interfering with the transfer of calcium into cells. Calcium plays an important role in muscle contraction. Decreasing the flow of calcium into cells causes the muscles in arterial walls to relax and expand. This results in improved blood flow to the heart and a reduction in the force needed to pump blood through the body. Individual CCBs may block calcium entry in slightly different ways, so the effects of each drug, both positive and negative, may vary.

Calcium channel blockers prescribed for the treatment of stable angina include amlodipine (Norvasc®), diltiazem (Cardizem®, Dilacor XR®, Tiazac®), and verapamil (Calan®, Covera-HS™, Isoptin®, Verelan®). Some of these agents may be given in combination with nitrates or beta-blockers for the treatment of stable angina. CCBs, but not beta-blockers, are used for the treatment of variant (Prinzmetal's) angina. Verapamil and diltiazem may be administered during acute coronary syndromes or following a heart attack if a patient is unable to take beta-blockers.

Some CCBs have the potential to weaken the heart's pumping action. In addition to relaxing the muscles in the arterial wall, these drugs affect the heart muscle and can reduce heart rate, which can be a problem in individuals with certain heart conditions. The most common side effects associated with CCBs are headache, low blood pressure, dizziness, edema (fluid retention), flushing, heart palpitations, and constipation.

ACE Inhibitors and Angiotensin Receptor Blockers (ARBs)

Angiotensin-converting enzyme (ACE) inhibitors and ARBs inhibit the *renin-angiotensin-aldosterone system*, which is primarily responsible for regulating blood pressure and water balance in the body. ACE inhibitors limit the production of angiotensin II, which results in a variety of effects, including increased dilation (widening) of blood vessels. ARBs block the receptors for angiotensin II, resulting in similar effects. Some patients with stable or unstable angina may be prescribed ACE inhibitors because large studies have shown that they offer long-term protection against cardiovascular disease.[2] ACE inhibitors are especially useful in preventing and treating failure of the left ventricle, the chamber of the heart responsible for pumping blood to the rest of the body. They are given as soon as possible following a heart attack to patients who have developed left ventricular dysfunction or failure or who are at high risk because of high blood pressure, diabetes, or kidney disease. ACE inhibitors have been found to improve survival after a heart attack. Some examples of ACE inhibitors include captopril (Capoten®), enalapril (Vasotec®), lisinopril (Prinivil®, Zestril®), perindopril (Aceon®), ramipril (Altace®, Tritace®), and trandolapril (Mavik®). ACE inhibitors may be prescribed indefinitely. A common side effect is a dry cough, which may occur in about 10 percent of patients. Other potential side effects include low blood pressure, elevated blood potassium levels, and worsening of certain kidney complications (although some evidence suggests that ACE inhibitors may be beneficial in patients with chronic kidney disease).

There is not the same level of evidence for the use of ARBs following a heart attack as there is for ACE inhibitors. ARBs are generally prescribed to patients who are intolerant of ACE inhibitors. They do not typically cause a dry cough.

Antiplatelet Drugs

When an atherosclerotic plaque ruptures, platelets, which are small cells carried in the blood, immediately collect at the site of injury. There they become activated by a protein called *thrombin* and begin connecting to each other to form a plug in the vessel wall in a process known as *platelet aggregation*. The activation of platelets releases additional proteins that draw more platelets to the site of injury, which soon becomes sealed off by a blood clot. Antiplatelet drugs work by blocking the various receptors that cause platelets to become activated.

Aspirin

Aspirin is commonly used to relieve minor aches and pains, but it also has many beneficial effects on the cardiovascular system. It prevents the formation of blood clots by inhibiting platelet aggregation. It also reduces inflammation and improves the health of arterial walls in people with atherosclerosis. Daily aspirin use is recommended for people who have had a heart attack, unstable angina, an ischemic stroke, or a transient ischemic attack (TIA) in order to prevent a recurrent event. Many patients with stable angina will be placed on daily low-dose aspirin, in addition to other medications. Aspirin has been shown to reduce the risk for heart attack and sudden death in people with stable and unstable angina; previous heart attack, stroke, or TIA; peripheral artery disease; or a previous percutaneous intervention. Aspirin is also given to individuals with acute coronary syndromes or strokes immediately after arrival in the hospital. In addition, large clinical trials indicate that in patients without cardiovascular disease, aspirin protects against heart attack in men and against ischemic stroke in women.[3] Men and women with a high risk of suffering a first heart attack or stroke are therefore often advised to take aspirin on a preventive basis, but low-risk, healthy individuals are generally not advised to do so.

The major side effect with aspirin is gastrointestinal bleeding and upset. There is also a small increase in the risk of hemorrhagic stroke. The risk of bleeding is related to the dose of aspirin. Although aspirin is not a prescription medication, you should always consult your doctor before taking it on a regular basis. Recommended daily doses are generally between 81 to 325 milligrams.

ADP Receptor Inhibitors

Clopidogrel (Plavix®), ticlopidine (Ticlid®), and prasugrel (Effient®) prevent platelet aggregation by blocking ADP receptors, which are involved in blood clotting. Clopidogrel is the most commonly used drug in this class. It is an oral medication that is often used in patients who are allergic to aspirin. It is also frequently used in combination with aspirin. Clopidogrel may be prescribed for daily use in patients who have suffered a recent heart attack or stroke, who have undergone percutaneous coronary intervention, or who have peripheral artery disease. It can help in preventing a future heart attack, stroke, or death. In the hospital it is often administered to prevent clotting in patients with unstable angina or a heart attack, often in combination with aspirin. The major risk with clopidogrel, as with many other drugs that interfere with the blood-clotting process, is *major bleeding*, or internal hemorrhaging that can sometimes be fatal.

Ticlopidine can be used to prevent repeat strokes or TIAs in people who are allergic to aspirin. However, it carries higher risks than clopidogrel and is seldom used unless the patient does not respond to clopidogrel treatment. Risks include an abnormally low white blood cell count, a rare blood-clotting disorder, and liver abnormalities. Your physician will monitor your blood count periodically if you are prescribed ticlopidine. Prasugrel is another recently approved drug in this class that can be used to prevent clotting in patients with acute coronary syndromes who are undergoing percutaneous interventions. It is generally viewed as being more effective than clopidogrel, but it also has an increased risk of causing major bleeding.

Cilostazol

Cilostazol (Pletal®) is used to alleviate intermittent claudication in patients with peripheral artery disease. It is one of the few drugs approved for this purpose. Cilostazol inhibits platelet aggregation and dilates blood vessels, and it can help people with peripheral artery disease to walk for longer distances. It may take two to three months before the positive effects of cilostazol become apparent. The most common side effects include headache, diarrhea, abnormal stools, heart palpitations, and dizziness. The headaches are generally mild to moderate and tend to disappear over time. Certain drugs may interact with cilostazol, as does grapefruit juice, which should be avoided. Another drug used to treat intermittent claudication is *pentoxifylline* (Trental®), which is not an antiplatelet agent. It works by decreasing the thickness of the blood. Treatment with cilostazol is considered preferable to pentoxifylline.

Glycoprotein (Gp) IIb/IIIa Inhibitors

Glycoprotein IIb/IIIa inhibitors are a type of antiplatelet drug that is administered intravenously in the hospital and for brief periods of time. In patients with acute coronary syndromes, Gp IIb/IIIa inhibitors have been shown to reduce the risk for death and heart attack. They are especially given to high-risk patients who will be undergoing coronary angiography or percutaneous interventions.

Anticoagulant Agents

At the same time that platelets are activated and begin to collect at the site of a ruptured plaque, a protein called thrombin is formed. Thrombin stimulates platelet activation, and it also generates *fibrin*, which binds to the growing clump of platelets. A blood clot, or thrombus, is produced as the fibrin binds the platelets tightly together. In general, anticoagulants, sometimes also called antithrombotics, interfere with the production or activity of thrombin, which prevents the activation of platelets and subsequent clot formation.

Heparin

Heparin may be administered to patients with acute coronary syndromes, heart attack, and ischemic stroke in order to prevent existing blood clots from growing and new ones from forming. It may also be used to prevent blood clot formation during an invasive procedure, such as percutaneous coronary intervention or bypass surgery. There are two forms of heparin. *Unfractionated heparin* is a naturally occurring substance that is extracted from pig intestines or cow lungs. It works by binding to a protein called antithrombin, which then inactivates thrombin and other proteins involved in blood clotting. The effects of unfractionated heparin can be difficult to predict, and its use requires careful monitoring with repeat blood tests. It is administered intravenously and is typically used for less than forty-eight hours, as the risk of developing an abnormally low platelet count increases if it is used for longer periods of time. *Low-molecular-weight heparins* (LMWHs) have been chemically processed and consist of molecules that are much smaller than those in unfractionated heparin. They are easily administered by injection and require less careful monitoring. They are also associated with a lesser risk of abnormally low platelets. In general, LVMHs are considered to be more convenient, safer, and more effective than unfractionated heparin. However, the effects of heparin can be readily reversed by administering another drug called protamine sulfate, whereas the effects of LVMHs cannot.

Thrombin Inhibitors

Thrombin inhibitors are a newer class of drug that is sometimes used instead of heparin. They are administered by injection and include bivalirudin (Angiomax®) and fondaparinux (Arixstra®). They are often used instead of heparin during percutaneous coronary interventions. A new oral thrombin inhibitor, dabigatran (Pradaxa®), was recently approved for the prevention of stroke in people with an abnormal heart rhythm called atrial fibrillation.

Warfarin

Warfarin (Coumadin®, Jantoven®) is the most commonly used oral anticoagulant in the United States. It is derived from coumarin, a chemical found naturally in certain plants. Interestingly, warfarin was initially marketed as a pesticide for rats and mice, and coumarins are still widely used as rat poison. Warfarin can be toxic to humans if ingested in large doses, far greater than the amount prescribed by physicians. As an anticoagulant, warfarin works by inactivating vitamin K in the liver, which interferes with the production of proteins needed in blood clotting. Warfarin is typically given to patients with artificial heart valves or atrial fibrillation. Patients are given warfarin following a heart attack if they have atrial fibrillation, heart failure, blood clots within the heart, or a history of blood clots in the veins or lungs.

Thrombolytic Therapy

Whereas antiplatelets and anticoagulants prevent existing clots from growing in size and prevent new ones from forming, thrombolytic therapy, also called fibrinolytic therapy, actually dissolves blood clots. Thrombolytic therapy is used in patients who have suffered an ST-elevation myocardial infarction (STEMI) or ischemic stroke. It may also be used in individuals with critical limb ischemia. The purpose of these drugs is to restore blood flow to the heart, brain, or limb in order to save as much tissue as possible.

For individuals with STEMI, thrombolytic drugs work best when administered within one hour after the onset of symptoms. For each hour afterward, blood clots become harder to dissolve, and after about six hours, the drugs are no longer effective. For individuals with ischemic stroke, thrombolytic therapy needs to be administered within three hours (at some hospitals, within four and a half hours) following the start of symptoms. Thrombolytic agents may be administered intravenously or by injection. Complications, including major bleeding and hemorrhagic stroke, can occur in a small percentage of patients undergoing thrombolytic therapy. Additional medications may be administered to prevent internal bleeding or to keep unclogged arteries from reclosing.

PERCUTANEOUS INTERVENTIONS

The term *percutaneous* refers to medical procedures that provide access to organs or tissues through a needle puncture in the skin. In terms of atherosclerotic disease, percutaneous interventions allow for the clearing of blood vessels throughout the body using a catheter inserted through the skin (see chapter 3 for more on cardiac catheterizations). They are considered less invasive than surgical procedures that require the opening of the body, typically done with a scalpel. Percutaneous coronary interventions (PCI) can be performed for the treatment of heart attack, unstable angina, or stable angina, depending on the degree of blockage and the presence of symptoms. Percutaneous interventions can also be performed on other arteries, including for the treatment of peripheral artery disease.

Percutaneous Coronary Intervention (PCI)

Since it was first performed in 1977, PCI, also known as percutaneous transluminal coronary angioplasty (PTCA), has become a very common procedure. PCI is generally considered to be the optimal treatment for STEMI if the hospital has the available facilities. It is recommended that individuals with STEMI undergo PCI within ninety minutes of arriving at the hospital.

PCI is an emergency procedure when it is performed on a patient undergoing a heart attack, but it can also be performed on an elective, scheduled basis. Patients with stable or unstable angina may undergo PCI if they have significant atherosclerosis in the coronary arteries. PCI can result in relief of angina, improved circulation, better ability to exercise, and better heart function, even at rest. It may also result in improved survival in some individuals, although it does not stop or reverse the atherosclerotic process. One study, called COURAGE, found that in patients with stable angina, PCI and optimal medical therapy were equally effective in preventing future cardiovascular events, although PCI was better at relieving angina.[4] Thus, some physicians may choose to treat patients with stable angina with medications first, before considering PCI. Lifestyle changes and risk factor modification, particularly with lipid-lowering therapies, are essential after undergoing PCI.

The major complication with PCI is blood clotting leading to a heart attack. Throughout the procedure, antiplatelet and anticoagulant drugs are administered to prevent this from happening.

The first percutaneous procedure developed was *balloon angioplasty*. With this procedure, an interventional cardiologist inserts a catheter through the femoral artery in the thigh, the radial artery in the wrist, or the brachial artery in the upper arm and directs it into the blocked coronary artery. The catheter carries a small balloon inside. Once the catheter is in position, the balloon is inflated in order to compress and split the atherosclerotic plaque while also stretching open the vessel wall (see figure 5.1). The procedure may be performed in multiple arteries if needed, and then the catheter is removed.

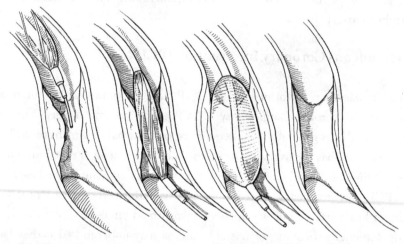

Figure 5.1. Clogged vessels can be reopened with balloon angioplasty. A tiny balloon, uninflated and inside a catheter, is positioned within an artery narrowed by atherosclerotic plaque *(second from left)*. The balloon is inflated *(third from left)*, which widens the artery *(right)*. *Illustration created by Herbert R. Smith Jr.*

In some cases, a separate procedure called *atherectomy*, may be performed in heavily blocked vessels to facilitate access prior to balloon angioplasty or stenting. With atherectomy, a tiny blade at the end of a specialized catheter is used to shave off bits of plaque, or a laser catheter vaporizes the plaque.

The majority of people who undergo angioplasty are now also treated with *stents*. With balloon angioplasty alone, *restenosis*, or the reclosing of a blood vessel after it has been unblocked, may occur in 30 to 60 percent of patients. Stents are thin mesh tubes made out of nickel and titanium that are inserted in arteries during PCI and left within the blood vessel permanently to prevent it from reclosing. They may also be inserted if an artery suddenly closes during balloon angioplasty due to a spasm. A collapsed stent is placed over a balloon catheter and positioned within the blocked artery. The balloon is inflated, which opens up the stent to its full size (see figure 5.2). Intravascular ultrasound may be used to assist the cardiologist in shaping the stent to the vessel wall. The catheter is withdrawn, and the stent remains in the artery.

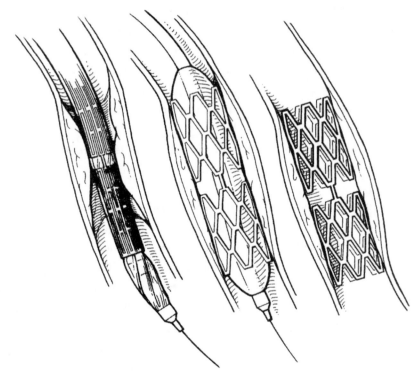

Figure 5.2. Stents are mounted over a balloon catheter and placed within the blocked artery *(left)*. The balloon is inflated, which expands the stent *(center)*. When the stent is in place, the balloon is deflated and withdrawn. The stent remains in the artery to keep it open *(right). Illustration created by Herbert R. Smith Jr.*

Even with stent placement, restenosis may still occur in 20 to 30 percent of patients. Restenosis occurs because balloon angioplasty and stent placement injure the tissues of the arterial wall, even as they allow for increased blood flow. The stent is perceived to be a foreign object and triggers an immune response, which causes scar tissue to grow near or inside the stent. As a result, the artery may narrow again, typically several weeks or longer after the procedure. *Drug-eluting stents* (DES), which were first introduced in the United States in 2003, are one of the most recent innovations in interventional cardiology to address this problem. They have a special coating that releases medication slowly over time directly into the arterial wall in order to prevent restenosis. Less than 5 percent of patients treated with drug-eluting stents experience restenosis. In the United States, the drugs first used for DES were paclitaxel, which is found in the bark of Pacific yew trees, and sirolimus, which is an antibiotic produced by soil bacteria. Newer agents, including a derivative of sirolimus called everolimus, are currently gaining in popularity. Many other agents are currently in development, and drug-eluting stents remain an area of intense investigation, testing, and research.

After PCI with or without stent placement, patients are generally discharged the following day if there are no complications.

Percutaneous Interventions for Peripheral Artery Disease

Percutaneous interventions and stenting can be performed for the treatment of peripheral artery disease, as well as for atherosclerotic blockages in the renal arteries feeding the kidneys and the carotid arteries in the neck. Patients with peripheral artery disease may be candidates for percutaneous interventions if they have severe symptoms of claudication, pain at rest, or tissue damage. Interventions at the iliac arteries in the pelvis have the best long-term success rates, with more than 60 to 85 percent of patients experiencing relief of symptoms even after five years. Interventions at the femoral artery in the thigh or the popliteal artery behind the knee may be successful in the short term, but long-term success rates decrease when procedures are performed farther down the leg.

SURGICAL INTERVENTIONS

As percutaneous interventions have become increasingly sophisticated and effective, the number of surgical interventions performed has decreased. Currently in the United States, PCI is performed approximately twice as often as the surgical procedure known as coronary artery bypass grafting (CABG). Surgery remains an important therapeutic option for many patients, however. Surgical techniques and technologies have evolved significantly over the past forty years that these procedures have been performed.

Coronary Artery Bypass Grafting (CABG)

Patients are carefully selected for surgical treatment based on the results of diagnostic tests to assess heart function (see chapter 3). Important factors that doctors consider are the site and extent of atherosclerotic plaque, the number of blood vessels affected, how well the left ventricle of the heart is functioning (as it is responsible for pumping blood to the rest of the body), and the patient's overall health. Patients with significant narrowing in the left main coronary artery in particular (greater than 50 percent) are likely to be recommended for surgery. The decision to undergo bypass surgery is made jointly by the physicians and the patient.

CABG is very effective in relieving the chest pain of angina, and it improves exercise capacity. It also improves long-term survival in patients with heart disease compared to the use of medication alone. Compared to PCI, CABG is about equally successful in the short term. CABG is considered preferable to PCI in patients who have more complex coronary lesions or plaques. The risk of surgery-related death or stroke is lower with PCI, but PCI is associated with more repeat revascularization procedures. With CABG, the risk of surgery-related death is about 1 to 2 percent. This risk is doubled or tripled in patients older than seventy years of age. In patients eighty years and older, the risk is 8 percent or more. The most common complication with CABG is the development of an abnormal heart rhythm called atrial fibrillation, which may occur in 25 to 30 percent of patients, particularly the elderly. Another complication is an inflammatory response that results from the surgery itself and from *cardiopulmonary bypass*, or the use of the heart-lung machine to replace the body's natural breathing functions during surgery. Drugs are administered before the operation to prevent complications such as blood clotting.

The bypass operation is performed under general anesthesia. During the operation, the heart is exposed by an incision made through the breastbone. In most cases, the patient is connected to the *heart-lung machine*, which allows the heart to be stopped and emptied of blood (see figure 5.3). The heart is stopped by clamping the aorta, the large artery that branches out from the heart, and by injecting a drug into the heart. The surgeon then creates "bypasses" around blocked sections of the diseased artery by attaching grafts that reroute blood flow (see figure 5.4). When all of these attachments are completed, the aortic clamp is removed, and blood flow through the coronary arteries begins to resume. In a few seconds, the heart starts to beat again. Sometimes the heart requires an electrical shock to produce a normal beating rhythm. Typically, patients stay in the hospital for four to seven days following CABG, unless there are complications.

In the past, a segment of the saphenous vein, a large vein in the leg, was used to form the bypass graft. More recently, heart surgeons have begun using the internal mammary artery, which runs down the rib cage just to the side of the breastbone, as the source for the graft. The internal mammary artery is especially resistant to atherosclerosis, and 80 to 95 percent of these grafts remain unblocked after ten years. Grafts may rarely be constructed from the radial artery in the forearm. Removal of portions of a vein or artery for grafts does not generally cause any circulatory disturbances since there are other blood vessels that take over instead.

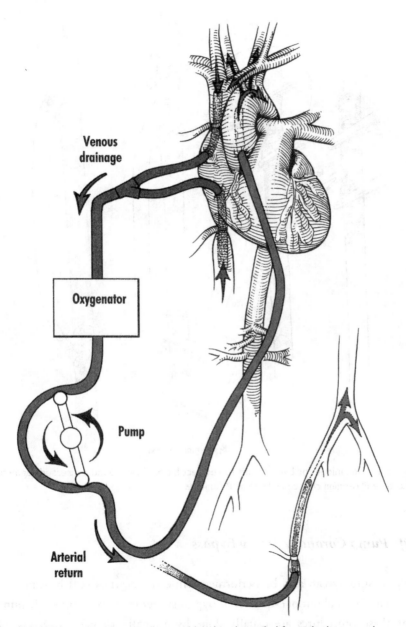

Figure 5.3. With cardiopulmonary bypass, blood is channeled from the heart to the heart-lung machine, which oxygenates the blood. It is then pumped back into the circulation. *Illustration created by Herbert R. Smith Jr.*

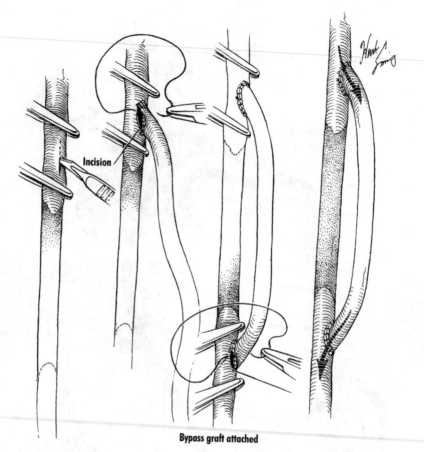

Figure 5.4. Technique for bypass graft to redirect blood flow around a diseased segment of artery. *Illustration created by Herbert R. Smith Jr.*

Off-Pump Coronary Artery Bypass

Bypass surgery can also be performed while the heart is still beating. It is estimated that about one-quarter of bypass surgeries are performed off-pump, but these procedures are usually done by a small group of surgeons who specialize in off-pump coronary artery bypass. It has not yet been definitively established how off-pump bypass and traditional CABG compare in terms of safety and efficacy.

Minimally Invasive Surgery

Minimally invasive coronary artery bypass surgery was first introduced in the mid-1990s and is still being evaluated. It uses much smaller incisions than in traditional CABG. Minimally invasive surgery decreases the length of hospital stays and the amount of hospital costs, but it may result in more complications than standard CABG. Minimally invasive surgery, or *port-access surgery*, is performed only at a few medical centers in the United States and requires a high level of skill. It involves exposing the coronary arteries through small incisions in the chest between the ribs, typically while the heart is still beating. In some cases, the surgeon looks directly at the area of operation. In others, small surgical instruments are inserted in the incision, and the procedure is viewed and performed with the aid of video monitors. Robots have been used to perform these technically difficult procedures, but the increased length of surgery with robots has so far limited their use.

Bypass Surgery for Peripheral Artery Disease

Bypass surgery can be performed to treat atherosclerotic blockages in the renal arteries of the kidney, the iliac arteries in the pelvis, and the femoral arteries in the thigh. As with percutaneous interventions, bypass surgery at the iliac arteries is the most successful in the long term. Success rates decrease with procedures performed below the knee. Bypass grafts may be constructed out of synthetic materials or from the saphenous vein in the leg.

Carotid Endarterectomy

Carotid endarterectomy is a surgical procedure used to prevent strokes in patients with extensive atherosclerosis of the carotid artery. It was first performed by one of the authors (MED) on August 7, 1953, at the Baylor College of Medicine and the Methodist Hospital in Houston, Texas. This procedure, which is typically performed under general anesthesia, involves making an incision in the neck to expose the blocked carotid artery (see figure 5.5). Clamps are placed on the artery around the area of blockage to prevent blood flow, and an incision is made in the artery. A small plastic tube is inserted to allow blood flow to the brain. Next, the atherosclerotic plaque inside the artery is peeled away from the vessel wall. After the plaque is completely removed, the artery is sewn shut, and the clamps are unfastened. The procedure takes about two hours and requires a hospital stay of one or two days. The major complication with carotid endarterectomy is suffering a stroke during the procedure; this risk is between 1 and 3 percent. Another potential complication is nerve damage to the neck, which generally disappears after a week or two.

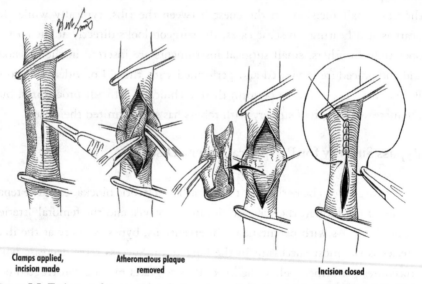

Clamps applied,
incision made

Atheromatous plaque
removed

Incision closed

Figure 5.5. Technique for carotid endarterectomy. *Illustration created by Herbert R. Smith Jr.*

CARDIAC REHABILITATION

With modern technological and medical advances, more people than ever before are surviving cardiac events. Cardiac rehabilitation is a process designed to minimize the physical and psychological effects of heart disease, return the patient to a full and productive life, restrict the progression of atherosclerosis, and reduce the risk for coronary death. It includes patient and family education, risk factor modification, and exercise training activities. Resumption of physical activity is essential to improving physical and emotional health, maintaining muscle tone and joint mobility, and preventing physical deconditioning associated with prolonged bed rest.

It is normal to feel apprehensive after suffering a heart attack, stroke, or other coronary event, or after undergoing cardiovascular surgery. Stress about being in the hospital, about suffering another coronary event in the future, or about how this event will impact your life can lead to a variety of emotions, including anxiety, depression, irritability, anger, fear, and a feeling of vulnerability. Community cardiac-rehab centers or hospitals often offer counseling and stress-management classes that can be beneficial to both the patient and his family. Education frequently gives people a sense of control and makes them feel more optimistic about the future. For most patients, irritability, fear, and depression will fade with time, usually after two to six months. If you or a cardiac patient close to you experience warning signs of serious depression (problems with sleep or appetite, extreme fatigue or lethargy, emotional stress, apathy, low self-esteem, and despair), consult a physician. While depression can be related to anxiety or feelings of loss of control, it can also be a side effect of medications used to treat cardiovascular problems, such as beta-blockers.

Traditionally, cardiac-rehab programs have been divided into three phases consisting of inpatient care while still in the hospital, a monitored or home exercise program combined with risk factor modification, and a long-term community-based or home exercise program. Programs are tailored to meet an individual's specific needs and health status. In recent years, changing patterns in medical insurance reimbursement have typically led to shorter hospital stays and earlier transitions to home exercise programs.

Inpatient Rehabilitation in the Hospital

Rehabilitation begins as soon as the patient is stable. A variety of diagnostic tests, such as echocardiography, electrocardiography, nuclear scans, cardiac catheterization, or exercise stress testing, may be ordered to help the physician determine the extent of damage to the heart and to plan the recovery process (see chapter 3). An important component of inpatient rehabilitation is education and counseling for both patient and family. Hospital staff members will provide detailed information about coronary disease management and teach the patient how to take his pulse, recognize important symptoms, and obtain emergency medical care. They will identify which activities are safe to do during the first few weeks of recovery, and they will discuss the patient's cardiovascular risk factors and any medications that have been prescribed.

Another important component of inpatient cardiac rehab is helping to progressively resume physical activity. *Early mobilization*, or getting patients out of bed and walking around, speeds the transition to normal daily activities and helps lessen feelings of anxiety and depression. A physical or occupational therapist may supervise simple range-of-motion activities, leading up to walking for increasingly longer periods of time and to climbing stairs. The cardiac-rehab staff will also work with the patient on performing basic self-care activities, such as showering.

Outpatient Cardiac Rehabilitation and Risk Factor Modification

Outpatient rehabilitation generally begins one to two weeks after hospital discharge, occurs three times per week, and may last for one to four months. The rehabilitation team will discuss appropriate types of exercise and correct exercise techniques. It will also provide instruction on how to check exercise intensity and monitor symptoms. The team will create an individualized exercise prescription, which specifies the duration, frequency, and progression of physical activity. The patient may be monitored during exercise with an ECG for an initial period of time. Some individuals with access to outpatient cardiac-rehab programs benefit from group exercise. Others may prefer to exercise alone and should consult their doctors before initiating home-based programs.

Patient education and counseling are other important components of outpatient cardiac rehab. Modifying risk factors and changing harmful health habits are crucial in improving recovery. Quitting cigarette smoking, limiting dietary fat intake, losing weight if necessary, and controlling high blood pressure and diabetes can help limit progression of atherosclerosis and decrease risk for future adverse cardiovascular events.

Long-Term Maintenance

After achieving the designated level of physical activity, maintenance becomes the primary goal of the exercise program. Daily walking is strongly encouraged. Most heart attack survivors are able to resume their previous activities within a few weeks or months. Since each individual's medical condition and personal situation is different, it is best to consult with a physician for specific recommendations about when to return to work, drive a vehicle, or engage in sexual activity. Exercise testing during outpatient rehab may provide useful information about when it is safe to engage in these types of activities again. In general, individuals can usually return to work within a few weeks, although people with physically strenuous jobs should wait longer. A waiting period of one week to one month is recommended before driving a private vehicle. Sexual activity may generally be resumed within one week to ten days. Patients who have undergone CABG should avoid heavy lifting for eight weeks.

***

The first five chapters of this book have focused on the development, prevention, and treatment of atherosclerotic vascular disease. The next three chapters will focus on other conditions that commonly affect the heart, including arrhythmias, heart failure, and valvular disease. Sometimes these conditions may develop due to the effects of coronary heart disease. Damage from a heart attack can lead to arrhythmias or heart failure, for example. They may arise independently because of aging and other factors; or one condition may lead to another, as when valvular disease leads to heart failure. The following three chapters will describe how arrhythmias, heart failure, and valvular disease can develop; the different forms they can take; and the cutting-edge strategies for treatment and management of these various conditions.

CHAPTER 6

ARRHYTHMIAS

I n an average lifetime, the human heart beats more than 2.5 billion times. Except when it slows down at night or speeds up with exercise or stress, the heart typically maintains a steady, constant rhythm. At times, however, an abnormal rhythm, or arrhythmia, can develop.[1] Many cardiac arrhythmias, such as an occasional skipped beat or heart palpitation, are common and generally harmless. Others are dangerous and can cause fainting, increase the risk of stroke, or lead to death within minutes if not treated immediately. Some arrhythmias that are potentially serious produce no symptoms, while others may significantly impact quality of life.

Cardiac arrhythmias become more common with age. They can be set off by extreme fatigue, physical exertion, emotional stress, cigarette smoking, heavy drinking, and ingestion of stimulants (such as caffeine, cocaine, or ephedrine-containing decongestants and dietary supplements). Conditions including congenital heart defects, imbalances of electrolytes (potassium, magnesium, and calcium), thyroid disorders, inflammatory diseases, and problems in the autonomic nervous system (which carries nerve impulses from the brain and spinal cord to the heart) can also increase the risk for arrhythmias.

The most important factor contributing to the development of arrhythmias is acquired heart disease. Coronary artery disease, heart attack, and high blood pressure all damage the heart, as can heart surgery and other invasive procedures. This damage results in scar tissue and areas of "dead" muscle that can affect the normal flow of electrical impulses in the heart and thus set off an abnormal rhythm. Before describing the different kinds of arrhythmias and how they are diagnosed and treated, let's discuss how the normal heartbeat is maintained and how it can be derailed to produce an arrhythmia.

191

HOW ARRHYTHMIAS ORIGINATE

The heart is divided into four chambers. Blood first flows into the upper chambers of the heart, or the *atria*. It then moves to the lower chambers, called the *ventricles*, where it is pumped out of the heart to the lungs and to the rest of the body (see figures 6.1a and 6.1b). A patch of specialized cells in the right atrium, called the *sinoatrial (SA)* or *sinus node*, acts as the body's natural pacemaker and is primarily responsible for maintaining the heart's regular beating rhythm. The cells in the SA node generate electrical impulses that race along an established route, triggering each of the heart's chambers to contract.

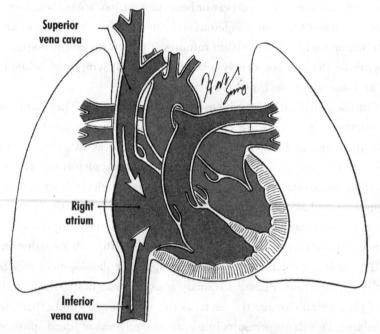

Figure 6.1a. Deoxygenated blood from the veins of the body enters the right atrium through the superior and inferior venae cavae and flows into the right ventricle. *Illustration created by Herbert R. Smith Jr.*

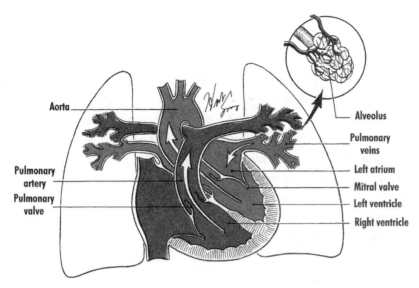

Figure 6.1b. From the right ventricle, blood is pumped through the pulmonary artery into the lungs, where it is oxygenated in the alveoli. The blood returns from the lungs through the pulmonary veins into the left atrium. After passing through the mitral valve, the blood is then pumped out of the left ventricle and into the aorta and the arteries of the body. *Illustration created by Herbert R. Smith Jr.*

Initially, a wave of electrical activity leaves the SA node and causes the atria to contract (see figure 6.2). It then travels to the heart's secondary pacemaker, called the *atrioventricular (AV) node*. As the impulse passes through the AV node, the ventricles fill with blood. The impulse then travels along a path of specialized cells called the "bundle of His" and divides into the left and right bundle branches. The bundle branches cause the ventricles to contract, pushing blood out of the heart and into the circulation. This entire process takes less than one second to complete. In an adult, the SA node normally fires an electrical impulse about sixty to eighty times every minute.

An arrhythmia can develop for one of three reasons: if the electrical impulses are emitted at the wrong time, if they are generated from the wrong place, or if they do not travel smoothly along their normal pathway. Some arrhythmias occur due to a combination of these factors. First, the natural pacemaker, the SA node, may fire too slowly or too quickly, producing a rhythm that may not be appropriate to the body's level of activity. Second, a group of cells other than the SA node can begin to send out electrical impulses and take over the heart's normal rhythm. Many cells in the heart are capable of acting as a backup pacemaker in case the SA node malfunctions, but this process can also occur at inappropriate times and produce an arrhythmia. Arrhythmias that arise because the SA node is not firing at the right speed or because a backup pacemaker has taken over the heart's normal rhythm are caused by disorders of *impulse formation*. Finally, some arrhythmias arise because of disorders of *impulse conduction*. Electrical impulses that are formed and sent out at the right time may slow down or completely stop as they travel to the ventricles. Or, in a process called *reentry*, they can get stuck in their usual pathway, detour into a bypass route, and then circle around and around along an abnormal circuit. When these kinds of deviations occur, the result is an arrhythmia.

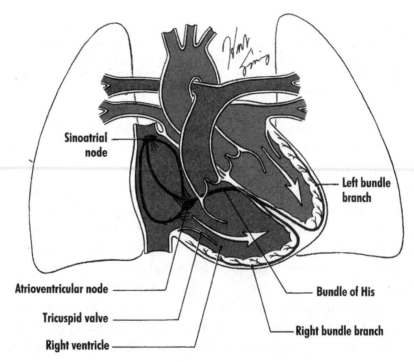

Figure 6.2. Electrical conduction system of the heart. *Illustration created by Herbert R. Smith Jr.*

TYPES OF ARRHYTHMIAS

Many arrhythmias pose no danger to your health. *Premature contractions* of the atria or the ventricles, which may feel like a skipped beat or heart palpitation, are very common and are often caused by external factors, such as smoking, drinking too much coffee, or consuming other stimulants. They are generally innocuous, but if they happen frequently or last for more than a few seconds, you may want to have your doctor check them out.

Sometimes the heart beats too slowly, too quickly, or unevenly. *Bradycardia* refers to a resting heart rate of fewer than sixty beats per minute, while *tachycardia* is the term used to describe a heart rate above one hundred beats per minute. The heart normally speeds up and slows down throughout the course of the day, but heartbeats that remain depressed or elevated for extended periods of time should be evaluated by a physician. Highly trained athletes are an exception since they may have very low resting heartbeats due to high cardiovascular efficiency. *Fibrillation* refers to uncoordinated, irregular contractions that do not effectively pump blood and that produce a "quivering" heart muscle.

Arrhythmias can start in different parts of the heart, and the places where they originate greatly affect their severity and recommended course of treatment. *Ventricular arrhythmias* are the most serious type of heart rhythm disturbance and demand immediate medical attention. Since the ventricles bear primary responsibility for pumping blood into the circulation, any significant dysfunction in these lower chambers of the heart can have serious consequences.

Tachycardia

Supraventricular or *atrial tachycardias* are fast heartbeats originating in the area above the ventricles either in the atria or AV node. They occur in many people and generally are not life threatening unless the heart is damaged in other ways. Supraventricular tachycardias may be associated with coexisting heart disease, and they may arise after a heart attack or heart surgery. There are numerous subtypes, including *paroxysmal atrial tachycardia (PAT)* or *paroxysmal supraventricular tachycardia (PSVT)*, in which arrhythmic episodes begin and end suddenly and are generally unpredictable. One type, called *Wolff-Parkinson-White syndrome*, is caused by abnormal electrical connections between the atria and the ventricles. Other atrial tachycardias often occur in people who drink excess caffeine or alcohol, smoke heavily, and are physically fatigued. In general, when the heart beats too rapidly, the ventricles do not have time to fill completely, which can compromise the heart's pumping ability. As a result, some people may experience symptoms such as dizziness or lightheadedness, heart palpitations, chest pain, or shortness of breath. Many patients do not require drug therapy, but for some types of atrial tachycardias, drug therapy or another form of treatment may be recommended if episodes are frequent and prolonged. A doctor may suggest vagus nerve stimulation (see the section in this chapter on diagnosing arrhythmias) or lifestyle changes such as consuming less alcohol, caffeine, and tobacco.

In *atrial flutter*, the atria may contract 250 to 350 times per minute, while the ventricles, unable to keep pace, contract about 150 times per minute. The heart's pumping efficiency declines, often leaving the person feeling weak or faint. Atrial flutter, an uncommon condition, is usually found in people with coexisting heart or valvular disease, recent heart attack or heart surgery, or chronic obstructive pulmonary disease. Many people with atrial flutter also have atrial fibrillation, which is a more common arrhythmia. With both conditions, blood pools in the atria because of ineffective pumping, which increases the risk that a blood clot will form and travel to the brain to cause a stroke. People with atrial flutter generally need anticlotting and antiarrhythmic medications. Cardioversion to restore a normal heart rate and catheter ablation to prevent recurrence may be recommended (see the sections in this chapter on cardioversion and catheter ablation).

Ventricular tachycardia originates in the lower chambers of the heart and can potentially lead to ventricular fibrillation, which is a life-threatening event. Ventricular tachycardia is strongly associated with coexisting heart disease, especially coronary artery disease, heart attack, and valvular dysfunction. It may develop in the days following heart surgery or a heart attack due to scarring or abnormal impulse conduction in the damaged area. In addition, many medical conditions, including infections, inflammatory or infiltrative disorders, and cancers that spread to the heart, can set the stage for ventricular tachycardia. Symptoms depend on the rate of the heartbeat (at least one hundred beats per minute at rest), the duration of episodes, and the presence of underlying heart disease. They range in severity from palpitations, breathlessness, fainting, or lightheadedness to dangerously low blood pressure, unconsciousness, and cardiac arrest. Some forms of ventricular tachycardia may be initially less dangerous if the heart rate is not extremely elevated and there is a measurable pulse. However, left untreated, ventricular tachycardia can degenerate into ventricular fibrillation. If you have palpitations, dizziness, near fainting, or chest pain, you should call 9-1-1 immediately. Immediate treatment of ventricular tachycardia may require intravenous medication and cardioversion, while long-term treatment to prevent recurrence may include antiarrhythmic medications, catheter ablation, surgery, or an implantable cardioverter-defibrillator (ICD, see the corresponding section in this chapter).

Fibrillation

Atrial fibrillation is one of the most common cardiac arrhythmias, particularly in people over the age of sixty-five. It affects approximately 2.2 million Americans and is more common in men than in women. It can occur in people with a variety of underlying heart, lung, or metabolic disorders, or it may arise in otherwise healthy individuals. Coronary artery disease, congestive heart failure, hypertension, valvular disease, and increasing age are common triggers, as are alcohol and caffeine. During atrial fibrillation, the upper chambers of the heart contract in an uncoordinated—and often very rapid—manner, so that the atria quiver without beating effectively. Electrical impulses transmitted through the AV node get out of sync, producing fast and highly irregular contractions of the ventricles. People with atrial fibrillation may have no symptoms, while others may experience heart palpitations, an uncomfortable and irregular thumping heartbeat, dizziness, sweating, fainting, chest pain, weakness, or a feeling of breathlessness.

An episode of atrial fibrillation is not immediately life threatening, but untreated atrial fibrillation can cause serious problems, including heart failure and stroke. Heart failure results when the chaotic contractions caused by atrial fibrillation are insufficient to sustain normal bodily functioning. The risk for stroke is increased because the atria do not empty properly when fibrillating, allowing blood to pool within the chambers and potentially clot. The clot can then travel through the circulation and cut off the flow of blood to the brain, causing a stroke. Atrial fibrillation is believed to be responsible for about 15 to 20 percent of all strokes, and people with atrial fibrillation are five to seven times more likely to suffer a stroke than people without atrial fibrillation. However, individuals younger than sixty-five years who do not have other risk factors for stroke, such as diabetes and high blood pressure, are at low risk for stroke. The population that is at the highest risk for stroke due to atrial fibrillation is elderly patients with diabetes, high blood pressure, or history of previous stroke. Thus, for patients with atrial fibrillation, it is very important to control risk factors for stroke such as hypertension, high cholesterol, and cigarette smoking (see chapter 2).

Patients may need to undergo transesophageal echocardiography in order to determine if there are any existing blood clots in the heart (see chapter 3). Anticoagulant medications are key to preventing strokes in patients with atrial fibrillation. In order to prevent new blood clots from forming, patients with atrial fibrillation are treated with anticoagulant drugs, primarily warfarin or newer oral medications like dabigatran (Pradaxa®) or antiplatelet agents like aspirin (also see chapter 5). Long-term treatment with warfarin has been shown to reduce the risk for stroke in patients with atrial fibrillation by as much as two-thirds. Warfarin is more effective than aspirin in the prevention of stroke, but it carries an increased risk of bleeding problems. Patients on warfarin are tested regularly to monitor the thickness or thinness of their blood and its tendency to clot, based on the International Normalized Ratio (INR). Warfarin dosages may change over time depending on the results of the INR. Consumption of foods containing vitamin K, such as green leafy vegetables and some vegetable oils, can cause INR levels to fluctuate. Antibiotics and multivitamins can also interfere with warfarin and affect INR levels. Dabigatran was approved in the United States in 2010 for the prevention of stroke in people with atrial fibrillation not caused by heart valve problems, and it does not require regular monitoring of INR levels.

Atrial fibrillation can be treated in several ways. One approach is to slow down the heart rate. During atrial fibrillation, the quivering contractions of the atria may reach rates of three hundred to six hundred beats per minute. The ventricles contract more slowly but still at an elevated rate of one hundred to one hundred sixty beats per minute. If left untreated, heart failure can develop, so medications such as beta-blockers, calcium channel blockers, and digitalis may be used to decrease the heart rate to less than eighty beats per minute at rest. Another approach is to use antiarrhythmic drugs to control the heart's rhythm and prevent episodes of atrial fibrillation from recurring. Antiarrhythmic drugs are effective only 50 to 70 percent of the time and can sometimes cause new arrhythmias (see the section in this chapter on drug therapies). Large clinical trials that have compared these two approaches to the management of atrial fibrillation (rate control versus rhythm control) have not found greater benefit with one strategy over the other, so patients are treated on an individual basis according to their symptoms.[2] If medications do not prove sufficient, other treatment options include cardioversion, catheter ablation, surgery, or pacemaker implantation (see the sections in this chapter on cardioversion and invasive interventions).

Ventricular fibrillation is a **medical emergency** that causes cardiac arrest and can lead to sudden cardiac death unless immediately treated. It is believed to be the major cause of sudden cardiac death and is most often associated with coronary artery disease. In ventricular fibrillation, muscles in the ventricles are reduced to rapid, erratic quivering and twitching. In this chaotic state, the ventricles lose their ability to pump blood out of the heart, leading to cardiac arrest. Without immediate intervention, blood flow to the brain stops, and sudden cardiac death follows. If someone suddenly collapses, becomes unresponsive, and stops breathing, they have gone into cardiac arrest. You should **call 9-1-1**, begin performing cardiopulmonary resuscitation (CPR) immediately if you are trained to do so, and use an *automatic external defibrillator* (AED) as soon as possible. CPR may be able to sustain a reduced level of cardiac output during ventricular fibrillation, but a defibrillator will be needed to "shock" the heart into a normal rhythm. AEDs can be found in many public places, often attached to walls, and most run with step-by-step, prerecorded voice instructions; they are designed to be used by laypeople who have received AED training. Long-term treatment for prevention of recurrent ventricular fibrillation may include antiarrhythmic medications or an implantable cardioverter-defibrillator.

Heart Block

In heart block, communication between the atria and the ventricles breaks down. The electrical impulses that originate in the SA node get delayed or stopped as they travel to the ventricles, disrupting the coordinated rhythm of the heart. Some forms of heart block produce no symptoms and do not require treatment; others can cause bradycardia, an extremely slow heart rate that can lead to lightheadedness, breathlessness, fatigue, weakness, and fainting. Many medical conditions are associated with heart block, including coronary artery disease and heart attack, inflammatory diseases, metabolic imbalances, infections, heart surgery, and tumors. In children, heart block may be present at birth. There are three designated degrees of heart block, ranging from first-degree heart block with no symptoms to third-degree (complete) heart block, in which no electrical signals from the SA node reach the ventricles. With complete heart block, backup pacemaker cells in the ventricles begin firing independently, but much too slowly. In such individuals, artificial pacemakers may be necessary to maintain a normal heart rate.

Sick Sinus Syndrome

Sick sinus syndrome, also known as sinus node dysfunction, refers to a group of abnormalities affecting the sinus, or SA, node. It is relatively uncommon and can be caused by damage to the SA node, scarring, and inflammation or degeneration of the nerves surrounding the node. Degenerative changes in the SA node become more common with age. In some patients, the heart may alternate between racing very quickly and beating too slowly. Sick sinus syndrome may also produce a variety of other rhythm abnormalities. Many people with sick sinus syndrome have no symptoms, while others may experience dizziness, palpitations, fatigue, nausea, or fainting. People with sick sinus syndrome who experience symptoms almost always need an artificial pacemaker, sometimes in addition to antiarrhythmic medication.

DIAGNOSING ARRHYTHMIAS

A thorough evaluation by a physician is essential in distinguishing between benign arrhythmias and those that are potentially lethal. Since arrhythmias may not always occur in the presence of a doctor, the information provided about prior episodes is crucial. If you experience an arrhythmia and seek medical attention, try to provide the physician with as much detail as possible. Questions you may want to consider are included in the following list.

- What were you doing at the time—lying down, watching a basketball game, pushing the lawnmower, arguing with a coworker?
- What do the irregular heartbeats feel like? Does your heart race, flutter, or skip a beat?
- When does the arrhythmia occur, and how long does it usually last?
- Do these abnormal heartbeats arise several times a day or just once in a while?
- Do they come and go suddenly or gradually?
- How do you feel during an episode? Does your chest hurt? Is it hard to catch your breath? Do you black out or feel as if you are going to faint?

The electrocardiogram (ECG) is the cornerstone of arrhythmia diagnosis. An abnormal pattern indicates a problem in a particular area or function of the heart and can, in some instances, provide enough information to establish a diagnosis. In other cases, twenty-four-hour ambulatory (Holter®) monitoring or an exercise stress test ECG may be necessary. If the origin of an apparently serious arrhythmia remains a mystery, or if the doctor needs more specific information before selecting a treatment, you may be asked to undergo extended cardiac event monitoring or electrophysiology testing (see chapter 3).

Coexisting cardiovascular diseases—and even some of the medications used to treat them—are common causes of arrhythmias. Noncardiac conditions such as thyroid disorders, inflammatory diseases, endocrine problems, or infections can also cause arrhythmias. In order to determine potential underlying causes of an arrhythmia, a physician will obtain a medical history, perform a physical examination, and may order blood tests. In addition, the doctor will ask about your use of caffeine, alcohol, cigarettes, decongestants, diet aids, and recreational drugs. If the arrhythmia is in progress, he may perform *vagal nerve stimulation*, usually with an ECG, to indirectly manipulate the vagus nerves, which help regulate heart rate. By gently massaging an area in the carotid arteries in the neck, the doctor may be able to slow your heart rate. Your heart's response to these maneuvers can provide important diagnostic information. Depending on the type of arrhythmia, the doctor may instruct you about other forms of vagus nerve stimulation (or "vagal maneuvers") to do at home, including holding your breath for a few seconds, dipping your face in cold water, or coughing.

TREATMENT FOR ARRHYTHMIAS

Treatment of heart rhythm disturbances can be complex. Sometimes more than one mechanism contributes to the irregular rhythm, and a two- or three-pronged therapy will be needed to address all the factors involved. Sometimes the medication given to correct one type of arrhythmia will worsen the condition or trigger another type of arrhythmia. In general, heartbeat irregularities arising in or involving the upper areas of the heart—supraventricular arrhythmias—are less serious and often respond well to medication. Ventricular arrhythmias—those originating in the lower chambers of the heart—can be quite serious and often require more complex interventions.

Drug Therapies

A wide array of medications is used to suppress heartbeat irregularities, although finding the most effective drug or the best dosage often requires experimentation and perseverance. Antiarrhythmic drugs are paradoxical in that they can both suppress and cause arrhythmias. The drug-induced arrhythmias may be harder to suppress or convert to a normal rhythm than the original arrhythmias and can even be potentially fatal. An individual's reaction to a particular medication can be unpredictable due to genetic differences or the coexistence of other heart problems. For these reasons, many doctors are turning instead to invasive interventions to treat arrhythmias such as catheter ablation, artificial pacemakers, and implantable cardioverter-defibrillators, which have become increasingly sophisticated and effective in recent years.

Antiarrhythmic drugs may have a variety of effects, including suppressing or altering the electrical impulses that control heart rhythm and rate, or reducing the heart muscle's response to these impulses. Some medications are given in intravenous form during an initial or life-threatening episode and may be continued in oral form after the heart rhythm has stabilized. Beta-blockers slow the transmission of electrical impulses from the SA node and through the AV node and are prescribed after a heart attack, when the damaged heart is likely to develop an abnormal rhythm. They may sometimes cause bradycardia, or a very low resting heart rate. Beta-blockers, including metoprolol (Lopressor®, Toprol-XL®), atenolol (Tenormin®), and carvedilol (Coreg®), are also used to treat atrial fibrillation and certain other supraventricular tachycardias. Some calcium channel blockers help control heart rate by damping the heart muscle's response to the erratic electrical impulses being transmitted. These agents, including verapamil (Covera-HS™) and diltiazem (Cardizem®, Dilacor XR®, Tiazac®), can be used to treat atrial fibrillation and supraventricular tachycardias. Some of the other medications that may be prescribed for certain types of arrhythmia include quinidine, flecainide (Tambocor®), propafenone (Rythmol®), amiodarone (Cordarone®), dronedarone (Multaq®), ibutilide (Corvert®), dofetilide (Tikosyn®), adenosine (Adenocard®), and digoxin (Lanoxin®). Ask your doctor for specific information about any antiarrhythmic medication you are prescribed.

Cardioversion

Cardioversion refers to the process of converting an arrhythmia back to a normal rhythm. It can be accomplished using some of the drugs listed above or by delivering an electrical shock to the heart at a specific point in the heartbeat. Cardioversion may be used to treat atrial fibrillation, atrial flutter, and ventricular tachycardia. When electrical shocks are delivered to an unconscious patient with ventricular fibrillation, the procedure is called *defibrillation*. Cardioversion is typically performed as a scheduled procedure on a patient who has been sedated. The shocks are administered through pads placed on the chest and/or back.

Invasive Interventions

Invasive treatments for arrhythmia have evolved dramatically in the past three decades and are now the treatment of choice for many conditions. Catheter ablation techniques have become increasingly refined, while pacemakers and implantable cardioverter-defibrillators have grown smaller in size, more responsive to the body's varying levels of activity, and more capable of sophisticated programming. For many patients, such procedures and devices provide a permanent solution to their heart rhythm abnormalities, although some patients may still require antiarrhythmic medications.

Catheter Ablation

Sometimes the best way to treat an arrhythmia is to deactivate the heart tissue responsible for causing the abnormal rhythm. Catheter ablation is a procedure that employs cardiac catheterization in order to deactivate a specific area of heart tissue (see chapter 3). A catheter is inserted in the femoral vein in the groin and directed to the cardiac chambers. An electrophysiology study is performed first in order to confirm the precise location of the heart tissue responsible for causing the arrhythmia. Radiofrequency energy, which is similar to the energy emitted by microwaves, is then directed through the catheter to destroy a small area of tissue using heat. During the procedure, the patient is awake, though sedated, and may feel some mild discomfort when the energy is applied. The entire procedure lasts from four to eight hours.

In the past, catheter ablation was performed using a direct electrical current, but radiofrequency energy is now generally used. In recent years, catheter ablation has also employed microwave energy and lasers, although less frequently. The use of lasers in particular continues to develop, as physicians and surgeons discover how best to incorporate this precise technology into delicate and complicated procedures. *Cryoablation*, or the use of very cold temperatures to deactivate tissue, is another variation on catheter ablation that has emerged recently.

Catheter ablation may be an option for individuals who do not respond to or cannot tolerate antiarrhythmic drugs or who prefer not to be on long-term drug therapy. It may be performed on patients with supraventricular or atrial tachycardias, atrial flutter, atrial fibrillation, and ventricular tachycardia. Success rates vary depending on the arrhythmia being treated and are improving. The risk of complications is relatively low. The most common risks include infection or bleeding. Sometimes catheter ablation can be unsuccessful if the exact source of the arrhythmia cannot be pinpointed. In less than 1 percent of cases, catheter ablation causes the heart to slow too much and necessitates the implantation of a pacemaker.

Surgical Treatment

As success rates with catheter ablation, artificial pacemakers, and ICDs have risen, the need for surgical treatment of arrhythmias has declined. Deactivation of the heart tissue responsible for producing an arrhythmia can often be accomplished less invasively through catheter ablation rather than surgery. Nowadays, surgical treatment of arrhythmias is most often performed if a person is undergoing open-heart surgery for another reason. Moreover, since many people with arrhythmias also have coronary artery disease, some may benefit from coronary artery bypass grafting (see chapter 5), which improves blood flow to the heart and reduces tachycardia.

Pacemakers

Artificial pacemakers have evolved from large, tabletop boxes resembling old-fashioned radios to sleek, metal-sheathed devices slightly larger than a quarter and weighing about one ounce. Modern pacemakers have a variety of programming options, and many can detect and respond to changes in body temperature, activity, oxygen consumption, and other measures. They contain microprocessors that record information about the heart's electrical activity and rhythm, and they can often transmit this information to doctors over the phone or Internet. Modern pacemakers can stimulate both the atria and the ventricles if necessary.

In the past, pacemakers were most often used to correct bradycardia, or a dangerously low heart rate. Now their use has expanded to people with difficult-to-control atrial fibrillation. In these individuals, the pacemaker acts as a backup or safety net in case the heart rate slows too greatly due to the effects of medication or catheter ablation. A temporary pacemaker may also be implanted after a heart attack, heart surgery, catheter ablation, or drug overdose to help maintain a normal heart rate while the patient is in the hospital. Some permanent pacemakers regulate the heart rate only if it falls or becomes irregular, while others operate continuously and change speed in response to the body's signals. Pacemaker implantation requires only local anesthesia and a mild sedative.

Pacemakers consist of a small metal case, which contains a battery and a generator that sends out electrical pulses, and one to three insulated wires with electrodes at their ends called leads. During pacemaker implantation, the leads are inserted through a large vein under the clavicle (collarbone) and directed into the heart. Pacemakers with one lead are called single-chamber pacemakers, and the lead is usually inserted in the right ventricle, which is the chamber of the heart responsible for pumping blood to the lungs for oxygen replenishment. Dual-chamber pacemakers contain leads in the right atrium, which receives deoxygenated blood from the body, as well as in the right ventricle. Newer triple-chamber pacemakers have leads in both ventricles and in the right atrium; these devices are used primarily for certain types of heart failure, and treatment is referred to as cardiac resynchronization therapy (see chapter 7).

When the leads are in place, they are connected to the pulse generator, which is typically implanted under the skin below the collarbone. The entire procedure usually takes between one and two hours. Patients typically stay in the hospital for one day, and the pacemaker is programmed using a computerized device. Patients may be asked to avoid heavy lifting or strenuous exercise for about one month, and there may be minor aches and pains at the site of pacemaker implantation. At hospital discharge, the doctor will provide advice regarding over-the-counter pain medications and return visits. After it has been established that the pacemaker is functioning normally, regular checkups will be scheduled; these may be in-person office visits, or information from the pacemaker may be sent over the phone or Internet. Pacemaker batteries typically last ten to fifteen years, and it is necessary to remove and reimplant the pacemaker in order to change the battery.

Potential problems in pacemaker placement include failure of the device to work properly: electrical impulses may fail to make the heart chambers contract, the sensors may not function accurately, the pacemaker may inadequately control the heartbeat, or the leads may become dislodged or may deteriorate. Other possible complications include infection, damage to blood vessels and nerves, and injury to the heart or lungs during the placement procedure.

In daily life, household appliances, including microwaves, are unlikely to interfere with a pacemaker, but patients should avoid holding electronic devices such as cell phones and portable music players over their pacemakers for extended periods of time. Pacemakers may set off metal detectors, although without affecting pacemaker function. Powerful electromagnetic fields caused by welding equipment and industrial power-generating equipment may interfere with pacemaker function. Patients should stand at least two feet away from such equipment and ask their physician about additional precautions to take. Patients with pacemakers are restricted from magnetic resonance imaging (MRI), although new MRI-compatible pacemakers are currently in development.

Implantable Cardioverter-Defibrillators (ICDs)

Before the advent of ICDs in 1980, most people who experienced ventricular fibrillation died of cardiac arrest unless they received emergency medical treatment within minutes. Now, patients can "carry" their own personal defibrillators, typically below their collarbone. ICDs are primarily used to treat people who have experienced ventricular tachycardia or ventricular fibrillation, but they can also be implanted in people who have weakened hearts due to heart attack or coronary artery disease, enlarged or thickened heart muscle (cardiomyopathy), or certain kinds of heart failure. ICD implantation is recommended to prevent sudden cardiac death in patients if they have severe left ventricular dysfunction, heart failure symptoms, and/or a history of brief episodes of ventricular tachycardia.

ICDs are implanted very similarly to artificial pacemakers and have a pulse generator and one to three leads. After implantation, the ICD is tested in the hospital with the patient under anesthesia. A typical hospital stay following ICD implantation is one to two days. People with ICDs need to take the same precautions regarding electrical devices as those with pacemakers. ICD devices typically last five to nine years.

An ICD continuously monitors the heart's rhythm, and when it detects an abnormality, it calculates the appropriate type of therapy. If the heart is beating too fast or too slow, it delivers small electrical impulses similar to a pacemaker to restore a normal rhythm. If the ICD detects ventricular tachycardia, it delivers a shock to the heart at a specific point in the heartbeat; the shock may feel like a thump in the chest that quickly dissipates. During ventricular fibrillation, the ICD delivers a high-energy shock to the heart. This process of defibrillation may feel like a kick in the chest, although ventricular fibrillation may cause the patient to lose consciousness prior to receiving the shock. There is no need for immediate medical attention if the patient feels fine shortly after receiving a shock. If she does not feel well after the shock, it may be necessary to call a doctor or an ambulance. Sometimes a patient may receive multiple shocks during a day, but frequent shocks over a short period of time indicate a need to seek emergency care to determine whether the device is malfunctioning or if the treatment, including antiarrhythmic medication, needs to be adjusted.

Having an ICD and receiving defibrillating shocks from time to time can be a stressful experience. Psychological counseling can help overcome the fear, anxiety, and depression that may complicate life with an ICD. These devices are standard treatment for people who have survived cardiac arrest or who are at high risk for cardiac arrest. It is important for the patient and the patient's family to know that with an ICD, the risk of sudden death from cardiac arrest is much lower than it would be with antiarrhythmic drug treatment alone.

CHAPTER 7
HEART FAILURE

Heart failure is a relatively common condition that occurs when the heart's ability to pump blood and/or its ability to relax between beats becomes impaired.[1] Although the heart continues to beat, it can no longer effectively propel blood to the lungs and to the rest of the body. Impaired heart muscle relaxation despite normal pumping function accounts for about one-half of all heart failure patients. Heart failure is one of the most frequent causes of hospitalization in the United States and is a major contributor to the cost of medical care.

Any kind of heart disease can lead to heart failure. Some people may be born with an abnormality that prevents the heart from functioning correctly. More often, conditions such as coronary artery disease or hypertension damage and weaken the heart over time, causing its pumping action to become increasingly less efficient. Damage to the heart valves or to the heart muscle itself can also cause heart failure.

Approximately 5.7 million people in the United States are living with heart failure, and approximately 670,000 new cases are diagnosed each year.[2] Like arrhythmias, heart failure becomes more common with age. In the United States, up to 10 percent of the population over the age of seventy-five is believed to suffer from heart failure, and about 80 percent of heart failure patients are over the age of sixty-five. Better treatment strategies are increasing life expectancy for people with coronary artery disease, but many of these patients will go on to develop heart failure as they age. Many heart failure patients require repeat hospitalizations, which is a major source of health care expenditures in the United States. Heart failure is the leading cause of hospitalization for individuals older than sixty-five years, with an average length of stay of five or six days.[3] According to the American Heart Association (AHA), a conservative estimate of the costs associated with heart failure in 2010, including health care services, medications, and lost productivity, is $39.2 billion.[4] Heart failure is a chronic condition that usually cannot be cured. But, with proper management including lifestyle changes and drug therapy, symptoms can be reduced, resulting in improved quality of life and decreased hospitalizations.

CAUSES AND CHARACTERISTICS

Heart failure is the inability of the heart to fully circulate the body with the oxygenated blood it needs. There are two general reasons why the heart typically fails. The first, called *systolic heart failure*, occurs when the heart is unable to contract fully and expel blood out into the rest of the body. Under normal conditions, as the volume of blood in the left ventricle (the chamber directly responsible for pumping blood to the rest of the body) increases, the heart compensates by stretching or increasing the length of the muscle fibers of the left ventricle. This results in a more forceful contraction, and the volume of blood expelled by the heart is increased. This principle is called the *Frank-Starling law of the heart*. When the stretching ability of the muscle fibers in the left ventricle begins to decrease, the contraction of the left ventricle is impaired, resulting in left ventricular dysfunction, and heart failure develops. The ejection fraction is a common measure used to describe the amount of blood that is pumped out of the ventricle with each heartbeat, and it is significantly reduced in patients with systolic heart failure. In an attempt to compensate for this reduced output, the heart may begin to beat faster, which can cause it to become further overworked. The heart may also compensate by enlarging over time.

The second general type of heart failure, called *diastolic heart failure* or *heart failure with normal ejection fraction*, occurs when the ventricles, or the lower chambers of the heart, are unable to relax and fill sufficiently with blood. People with diastolic heart failure may have a normal ejection fraction, but they experience other symptoms and signs of heart failure. The terms *systolic* and *diastolic* are also used in reference to blood pressure. *Systole* is the period of time during which the heart contracts, while *diastole* refers to the pauses between contractions when the ventricles fill with blood (see figure 7.1). Many people with heart failure have combined systolic and diastolic heart failure: there is both reduced blood flow into the ventricles and reduced force in pushing blood out into the arteries.

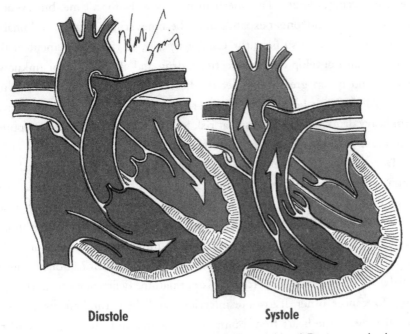

Diastole   **Systole**

Figure 7.1. During diastole, the heart relaxes and fills with blood. During systole, the heart contracts to pump blood to the body. *Illustration created by Herbert R. Smith Jr.*

One of the most common causes of heart failure is atherosclerotic disease, which usually results in combined systolic and diastolic heart failure. When the arteries become blocked due to atherosclerosis, reduced blood flow can deprive the heart of oxygen and nutrients, resulting in ischemia. The heart may become progressively weaker and unable to contract maximally as a result. Ischemia also causes the heart to become stiffer and prevents it from relaxing fully in between beats. Heart failure as a result of ischemia can happen gradually over time, but it can also develop suddenly. During a heart attack, blood flow to the heart is interrupted, which can create patches of dead tissue that are unable to contract at all. The stiff scar tissue that forms after a heart attack can further limit blood flow into the ventricles.

Hypertension is a frequent cause of diastolic heart failure, although it can also weaken the heart's ability to contract. When a person develops hypertension, the pressure within the blood vessels increases, which makes it more difficult for the heart to pump blood through the circulation. To compensate, the heart becomes larger. This mechanism may work for a time, but eventually the heart can no longer expand, and it becomes stiffer, weaker, and unable to contract and relax sufficiently. *Cardiomyopathy*, or the enlargement of the heart, can also develop due to infections, drug and alcohol use, or unknown reasons, and it can greatly hamper the heart's ability to relax and fill with blood. Alcohol can be toxic to the heart in excessive quantities, and long-term heavy drinking puts a person at risk for *alcoholic cardiomyopathy*. Stopping drinking is essential for successful treatment.

Heart failure can develop due to a variety of other causes. In general, any kind of damage to the heart can lead to heart failure, but in some cases, the cause of heart failure may be unknown or may be genetic in origin. Diseases of the valves that regulate blood flow into and out of the heart, arrhythmias, severe lung disease, inflammation of the heart muscle (myocarditis) or of the sac surrounding the heart (pericarditis), birth defects, chemical or hormonal imbalances in the blood, hyperthyroidism, thiamine deficiency, chemotherapy drugs for cancer, other diseases or infections, and the natural effects of aging can all prevent the heart from pumping efficiently and can possibly lead to heart failure. During the mid-1960s, beer containing cobalt to stabilize foam caused outbreaks of severe heart failure; after identifying the cause, cobalt was removed from the brewing process, and no more episodes were reported.

Doctors sometimes distinguish between *left-sided* and *right-sided* heart failure. The left side of the heart is responsible for pumping oxygen-rich blood to the rest of the body, while the right side pumps oxygen-depleted blood to the lungs for replenishment. Many people initially have left-sided heart failure, which is the more common of the two conditions, but may go on to develop right-sided failure in addition. Another distinction is between *chronic* and *acute* heart failure. Heart failure is generally a chronic condition, but sometimes the symptoms of heart failure can develop suddenly or become rapidly more severe. Acute heart failure, in which symptoms become severe over a short period of time, is not the same as a heart attack or as cardiac arrest, which occurs when the heart stops beating entirely.

The primary symptoms of heart failure are fatigue or weakness, difficulty breathing, and swelling, particularly in the lower body. Fatigue and weakness occur because the skeletal muscles are not receiving sufficient oxygen-rich blood. This lack of oxygen may cause feelings of faintness or dizziness, and it can affect the ability to exercise. Shortness of breath, called dyspnea, may also make it more difficult to exercise. Shortness of breath occurs when the left ventricle is unable to expel enough blood, so that blood coming into the left side of the heart from the lungs gets backed up, causing fluid to leak back into the lungs. As heart failure worsens, feelings of breathlessness may become more troublesome and may occur not only during exercise, but also while lying down, sleeping, or at rest. Sometimes elevating the head while lying down will improve symptoms. In more severe cases, patients may wake up suddenly at night with a suffocating and anxious feeling and have to sit bolt upright in bed for thirty minutes or longer before they can fully regain control of their breathing; these attacks are referred to as *paroxysmal nocturnal dyspnea*. A dry, hacking cough and wheezing are other symptoms of heart failure that develop when fluid backs up in the heart and begins to leak into the lungs. Of course, symptoms like fatigue, weakness, breathlessness, and coughing can also occur for many other reasons besides heart failure and should always be evaluated by your physician.

Swelling is often the symptom that sends patients to the doctor. Fluid accumulation in the body's tissues, called edema, occurs when the heart fails to pump blood forcefully enough to keep the circulation flowing properly. In addition, the kidneys receive less blood and become less able to flush sodium and water out of the body. As a result, fluid begins to seep from the blood vessels into body tissues and cavities. Gravity tends to pull fluid downward into the feet and ankles (see figure 7.2). Swelling in the legs can also be caused by slow blood flow in the legs due to extended periods of immobility, such as a long airplane flight or prolonged bed rest. Heart failure can addition-ally cause fluid to collect in and around the lungs, which is called *pulmonary edema*. When fluid invades the lungs and also causes swelling in the legs and ankles, the condition is called *congestive heart failure*. Sometimes this term is used interchangeably to refer to heart failure in general.

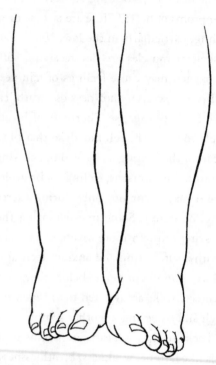

Figure 7.2. When heart failure causes fluid retention, the feet, ankles, and legs may swell. *Illustration created by Herbert R. Smith Jr.*

Other symptoms of heart failure include nausea or lack of appetite caused by increased fluid around the stomach and intestines, a confused mental state due to poor blood flow to the brain, and an increased heart rate. Some people with mild heart failure may experience no symptoms at all.

DIAGNOSIS AND MANAGEMENT

To understand the reason a patient is experiencing shortness of breath, fatigue, and swelling, a physician will obtain a medical history, perform a physical examination, and order other studies, such as a chest x-ray, echocardiography, electrocardiography, blood tests, nuclear imaging, and exercise stress testing (see chapter 3). Individuals with heart failure often have a third or fourth heart sound—extra heart sounds that occur in addition to the normal two heart sounds ("lub-DUB"). The third heart sound can sometimes be heard in children and adults younger than forty years, but it is rare in healthy adults above that age. A fourth heart sound is always abnormal. In a person with heart failure, increased pressure in the right ventricles can cause the jugular veins in the neck to become distended. A doctor may order a chest x-ray to see if the heart is enlarged or if the lungs are congested. The ejection fraction, or pumping function of the heart, and the extra heart sounds can be evaluated with echocardiography, while an electrocardiogram (ECG) can indicate whether an arrhythmia may play a role in heart failure. Blood tests—including measures of hemoglobin; electrolytes; and liver, thyroid, and kidney function—can help establish a diagnosis of heart failure and identify other coexisting diseases. Sometimes the symptoms of heart failure can be caused by anemia or by dysfunction of the liver or thyroid. In patients with severe heart failure, the liver can become enlarged and tender as blood builds up inside it. In very severe cases of liver enlargement, a patient may develop jaundice (yellowing of the skin and whites of the eyes). Finally, nuclear-imaging tests provide information on how well the ventricles are functioning when the heart contracts; echocardiography and nuclear imaging may be combined with exercise testing to compare the heart's performance at rest and during exertion.

Heart failure is classified into four categories based on a system established by the New York Heart Association. This system is often used by physicians to determine the course of treatment. It classifies heart failure patients according to how they feel their symptoms impact their daily activities and quality of life. Class I heart failure is associated with no symptoms or limitations on physical activity; class II is characterized by mild symptoms, such as shortness of breath, fatigue, and heart palpitations, during moderate activity. With class III, or moderate heart failure, ordinary activity becomes limited because of symptoms, and the patient is only comfortable at rest. Patients with class IV, or severe heart failure, are unable to engage in any physical activity without discomfort, and they experience symptoms even while resting. Patients with mild heart failure may require no medical treatment other than following heart-healthy dietary guidelines and exercise recommendations. Patients with severe heart failure may require both medical and surgical treatment.

Lifestyle Changes with Chronic Heart Failure

Dietary and other lifestyle changes are important in treating chronic heart failure. Dietary changes aim to reduce the workload of the heart, regulate fluid intake, and improve overall nutrition. Being overweight increases the strain on the heart, which is forced to work harder in order to pump blood to excess body tissues, so it is important to reach and maintain an optimal weight. Weight reduction is especially important in patients with high cholesterol or triglycerides, high blood pressure, coronary artery disease, or other risk factors for cardiovascular disease.

Controlling sodium intake helps to prevent the symptoms of heart failure from worsening. When heart failure slows the circulation, the kidneys are unable to effectively clear the body of excess fluid and sodium, so patients may be asked to restrict sodium consumption. People with heart failure often experience an intense thirst, but may be asked to limit daily fluid intake to prevent swelling. Limiting alcohol is recommended because it can damage the heart wall and cause arrhythmias, and coffee should be avoided or consumed in moderation. Smoking should be abandoned immediately because it makes breathing more difficult, and it impedes blood flow in the arteries surrounding the heart, thereby worsening the symptoms of heart failure.

Patients with heart failure should strive to achieve a balance between rest and physical activity. After acute heart failure, some bed rest is essential, but it is important to get moving again early in treatment. Walking or biking around the neighborhood can improve spirits as well as the cardiovascular system. Swimming spares the bones from jarring contact with pavement, while gardening may be a good way to transition from rest to a higher level of activity. Finding the right pace for an activity and building on it are fundamental to improvement. In addition, it is advisable to get vaccinations for the flu and for pneumonia in order to reduce the risk for lung infections.

Heart failure can greatly affect quality of life. Patients may have to make significant changes in their lifestyles and take a variety of medications. Multiple hospitalizations over time are common, particularly in the elderly. If you have heart failure, enlist family and friends in your treatment so that they can support you in your effort to live as fully as possible within the confines of your illness. You may also want to seek the help of a professional counselor, social worker, or support group, all of which can assist you in examining your feelings regarding your diagnosis and treatment, as living with heart failure can be stressful at times.

Although it may be unpleasant to think about, plan what you would do in the event of an emergency. Talk to your attorney, your family, and your health care team about how to make decisions about your medical care through advance directives.

Drug Therapy

Many patients with chronic heart failure will be advised to begin a combination of diet modification and drug therapy. Traditionally, medications for heart failure have been prescribed to reduce swelling and fluid buildup (diuretics), to relax blood vessels and improve blood flow (vasodilators), and to strengthen heart function. There are also newer classes of medications, including ACE inhibitors, angiotensin receptor blockers (ARBs), and beta-blockers, which work by interfering with various hormonal systems that become activated as the heart begins to fail. These newer drugs are now used regularly in most patients with heart failure, as they have been shown to improve survival. Many of the medications for heart failure are also used to treat other heart conditions and are discussed in chapters 2, 5, and 6.

Angiotensin-converting enzyme (ACE) inhibitors are often prescribed for hypertension because they act as vasodilators to expand blood vessels, but they have additional beneficial effects in patients with heart failure. By inhibiting the production of angiotensin II, ACE inhibitors act to reduce fluid and salt retention, relax blood vessels, and prevent the heart from enlarging. They may also prevent the development of heart failure in patients who have sustained damage to the left ventricle after a heart attack. A dry cough is a common side effect, and patients who cannot tolerate ACE inhibitors may instead be prescribed an ARB, which has similar beneficial effects but does not cause coughing. Common ACE inhibitors used for heart failure include captopril (Capoten®), enalapril (Vasotec®), lisinopril (Prinivil®, Zestril®), ramipril (Altace®, Tritace®), quinapril (Accupril®), and trandolapril (Mavik®). Candesartan (Atacand®), losartan (Cozaar®), and valsartan (Diovan®) are commonly prescribed ARBs that have been extensively studied in patients with heart failure.

Beta-blockers are used to slow down the heart and decrease its contractile strength in patients with coronary artery disease. These changes can improve heart function over time. They work by inhibiting a complicated system of hormones and nerves, and they also act on genes in the heart to improve its function and prevent it from enlarging. Beta-blockers have been found to greatly improve survival in patients with heart failure, and most patients will be prescribed one in addition to an ACE inhibitor, generally in a low dose that is gradually increased over a period of time. Common and well-studied beta-blockers for treatment of heart failure include bisoprolol (Zebeta®), carvedilol (Coreg®), metoprolol (Lopressor®), and nebivolol (Bystolic®).

Along with restricting sodium and fluids in the diet, doctors may prescribe diuretics to help patients reduce the sodium and fluid in their bodies through increased urination. Diuretics, which are also commonly used to treat high blood pressure, can reduce swelling in the ankles and legs and make it easier to breathe deeply. Doses for heart failure are generally higher than those prescribed for hypertension. Doses that are too high may cause tiredness and fatigue in elderly individuals. Patients with severe heart failure are often prescribed loop diuretics, whereas those with milder cases may receive thiazide diuretics. A third type, potassium-sparing diuretics, help reduce fluid retention without decreasing potassium levels in the body and are most often paired with one of the other two types of diuretic. Two potassium-sparing diuretics called spironolactone (Aldactone®) and eplererone (Inspra®) act by interfering with the hormonal system that controls water and sodium reabsorption, and these two drugs in particular have recently been shown to improve survival in systolic heart failure patients. Many other diuretics may also be prescribed.

While many heart failure patients will have improved symptoms when taking a combination of ACE inhibitors, ARBs, beta-blockers, and diuretics, other patients may need additional drugs. Vasodilators, including oral nitrates, which are used primarily for the treatment of angina, and hydralazine may help improve blood flow through vessels. In the African American Heart Failure Trial, which included patients with advanced heart failure who identified as African American, the addition of the nitrate drug isosorbide dinitrate and the vasodilator hydralazine to standard medical treatment was found to reduce mortality by 43 percent, decrease hospitalizations, and improve quality of life compared to standard treatment alone.[5] This drug combination, available commercially as BiDil®, is now recommended for self-identified black patients with symptomatic systolic heart failure receiving optimal medical therapy; its effects on nonblack patients remain unclear. In the past, digoxin or digitalis, a drug that increases the contractile force of the heart and slows the heartbeat, was considered the primary treatment for heart failure, although it can be toxic and requires careful monitoring. Digitalis was originally made from the dried leaves of foxglove plants and can alleviate the symptoms of heart failure, although it has not been shown to reduce the risk for death. With the development of newer, more effective drugs, the use of digoxin has decreased substantially, although specific patients may benefit from treatment. There are also a variety of additional drugs that can be administered intravenously if necessary.

Device and Surgical Therapies

In some patients, the underlying cause of heart failure can be treated surgically. If heart failure is the result of dysfunctional heart valves, surgery to repair or replace them can be performed (see chapter 8). Some patients who have developed heart failure due to coronary heart disease may benefit from coronary artery bypass graft (CABG) surgery or percutaneous coronary intervention, both of which can help restore the flow of blood and oxygen to nutrient-depleted heart tissues (see chapter 5). Surgical removal of scar tissue and other abnormalities of the heart muscle, whether present at birth or acquired later in life, may also be a possibility.

New surgical techniques for heart failure are currently under investigation. These procedures aim to prevent the enlargement of the heart and to reduce tension within its walls, and they can involve placing a patch on the left ventricle, enclosing the heart in a mesh bag, or compressing the walls of the left ventricle with polyester tension rods. These approaches have shown initial promising results, but they are considered experimental and may not be available except to participants in clinical trials. One surgical procedure that has been performed in limited numbers since the mid-1980s, called *dynamic cardiomyoplasty*, involves wrapping the heart with the patient's own skeletal muscles, most commonly the latissimus dorsi from the back, and stimulating contractions with a specialized pacemaker. A newer approach derived from this procedure is *cellular cardiomyoplasty*, in which individual stem cells are injected into the damaged heart tissue to strengthen its contractions. It may be that the future treatment of advanced heart failure may lie in stem cell therapy, which could theoretically lead to the generation and growth of new heart tissue (see chapter 9).

If the underlying cause of heart failure cannot be addressed surgically and if medication does not sufficiently alleviate symptoms, it may be necessary to use mechanical devices that assist the circulation or to evaluate the feasibility of heart transplantation. Since it was first performed in 1967, heart transplant has traditionally been the only option available for individuals with severe heart failure. However, the number of heart donors per year is only about four thousand worldwide. Over the past decades, mechanical devices that can prolong life in individuals awaiting transplant or that can even be used on a long-term or permanent basis have been developed. These devices have become increasingly smaller and more portable, and doctors have become considerably more knowledgeable about how to insert and maintain them.

Assisted Circulation

Patients may need mechanical support if their blood pressure falls to life-threateningly low levels or if vital organs become endangered by lack of blood flow. Some patients require temporary assistance in order to give their hearts time to recover after a heart attack or surgery, while others may need a ventricular assist device (VAD) as a *bridge-to-transplant therapy* as they await a donor organ. Still others may not be candidates for heart transplant, and a VAD may be inserted as *destination therapy* (intended for long-term, permanent use).

The *intra-aortic balloon pump*, first developed in 1961, is one of the most commonly used forms of short-term mechanical assistance. It is placed in the aorta through a catheter, which may be inserted through the femoral artery in the groin or the axillary artery in the upper arm. It consists of a helium balloon that is alternately inflated and deflated by a bedside machine. The timing of inflation and deflation is coordinated with the heartbeat so that blood moves forward through the aorta with greater ease and less effort is placed on the heart. The pump also helps to increase blood flow to the brain, the kidneys, and the heart itself. It is most often used in patients with severe heart failure or shock following a heart attack, and it can also be used to support the heart during percutaneous coronary intervention. It is a temporary device that is generally only left in for a few days, and it requires patients to be immobilized in bed.

Ventricular assist devices developed from the heart-lung machines that are used during open-heart surgery. In the hospital, similar machines are used for short periods of time (generally less than one week) to provide mechanical support to the circulation while allowing the heart time to recover enough strength to beat on its own. In addition to external devices used in the hospital, ventricular assist devices can be partially or totally implantable. The first left ventricular assist device (LVAD) was temporarily implanted by one of the authors (MED) in 1963. Since then, smaller devices capable of longer use have been developed, and many are based on Dr. DeBakey's original model. Unlike the intra-aortic balloon pump, which helps increase the flow of blood as it travels its natural route through the heart, VADs draw blood out of the lower ventricles of the heart through a tube and then pump it mechanically back out into the aorta. VADs can provide assistance to the left or right ventricle, or both.

Pulsatile devices mimic the normal heartbeat, with contractions followed by brief pauses, and they generate a pulse in the patient using one. For example, the HeartMate® by Thoratec is available in the United States as a bridge-to-transplant therapy and as permanent destination therapy. These devices are portable and can enable patients to move around relatively normally. The pumps and the tubes that circulate blood are implanted in the chest, and another tube goes through a hole in the abdomen to connect to an external battery pack that is worn around the waist. Thoratec has another device in which the pumps and battery pack are carried outside the body, connected to a tube that is then attached to the heart.

In 2001, the results of a major study called REMATCH, which included 129 patients with severe heart failure who were not candidates for heart transplant, showed that the HeartMate significantly improved survival and quality of life compared to treatment with drugs alone.[6] In this study, one-half of the patients who received a VAD survived after one year, compared to only one-quarter of patients who received medication alone. Since this trial, VADs have become accepted as a permanent treatment alternative in patients not eligible for a transplant.

While it is clear that the most severely ill patients benefit from a long-term VAD, it has not yet been established whether the use of long-term or permanent devices should also be extended to individuals who may not have such greatly decreased life expectancy. Newer and more sophisticated devices, which are designed to overcome many of the problems that have traditionally limited the use of VADs, continue to be developed and tested. For example, one potential risk is blood clotting, which can occur whenever blood comes into contact with a foreign body; therefore, many patients need to take anti-clotting drugs. Newer devices, including the HeartMate, are constructed of special materials to minimize clotting. Pulsatile devices are also relatively large and cannot be implanted in younger children and smaller patients. In addition, they have many moving parts that require a constant supply of energy and tend to malfunction after a period of time. Finally, VADs in general pose a high risk for infection and require the use of antibiotics.

The next-generation VADs currently being tested include totally implantable pulsatile devices and devices incorporating new kinds of pumps that move blood flow continuously through the body without generating a pulse. These pumps are smaller, easier to implant, and have lower energy requirements. One of these is the MicroMed HeartAssist 5®, originally designed by one of the authors (MED) and Dr. George Noon of Baylor College of Medicine in conjunction with NASA/Johnson Space Center. This cylindrical titanium device is three inches long and about one inch in diameter and weighs only a few ounces. It is currently approved in the United States for use in children aged five to sixteen years, and testing in adults is underway.

Cardiac resynchronization therapy (CRT), also known as *biventricular pacing*, describes treatment with a special kind of pacemaker that is connected to both ventricles and to the right atrium of the heart (see chapter 6). It is used in patients with moderate or severe systolic heart failure who do not respond to medication and whose ventricles do not contract at the same time. As with a regular pacemaker, small electrical impulses are transmitted to the heart to trigger contractions. The left and right ventricles are stimulated to contract at the same time, improving overall heart function. The device can also incorporate a defibrillator if necessary. Studies have shown that biventricular pacing can improve symptoms and quality of life, reduce hospitalizations and mortality, and reverse heart-failure-induced enlargement of the ventricles.[7] However, the therapy has no effect on symptoms in approximately one-third of treated patients.

Total artificial hearts (TAH) are used only in a small number of patients. There are currently two types of artificial heart available in the United States. The CardioWest™ temporary TAH was approved in 2004 for hospitalized patients with severe heart failure awaiting a transplant. Fewer than seven hundred of these devices have been implanted since that time. In 2006, under a Food and Drug Administration Humanitarian Device Exemption, the AbioCor® TAH was approved for use in patients dying of heart failure who are not candidates for a transplant. (A Humanitarian Device Exemption can be applied to devices that may be used to treat fewer than four thousand people in the United States per year.) Both devices are similar, except that the CardioWest TAH is connected through a hole in the abdomen to a large machine. The AbioCor TAH is fully implanted in the body, and the battery is charged through the skin with a magnetic charger. Risks associated with total artificial hearts, which greatly limit their use, include blood clotting, infection, bleeding related to the implantation surgery, and device malfunction.

Heart Transplantation

Transplantation of the heart is a dramatic means of treating carefully selected patients with profoundly severe heart failure. Approximately 80 percent of patients with severe heart failure treated with medications alone die within two years. In contrast, the survival rate in patients receiving a heart transplant is about 85 percent after one year and slightly less after two years. Of the approximately seventy-eight thousand patients worldwide who have reportedly received a heart transplant between 1982 and 2007, one-half survive longer than ten years. About 20 percent remain alive twenty years post-transplant.

The demand for donor hearts far exceeds supply, and the sickest patients are the ones most likely to be selected for heart transplant. Most patients who are transplant candidates have not responded to aggressive drug treatment, have required repeated hospitalization to manage heart failure, and may be dependent on intravenous medications or mechanical assistance to support the heart. Among patients who are not bedridden, only those with the least chance of survival without a transplant are considered to be candidates for a transplanted heart. Potential candidates are carefully screened and undergo numerous tests. In the past, individuals over the age of sixty-five years were not considered transplant candidates, but most transplant centers are now more flexible regarding age, provided the patient does not have other conditions that would prevent her from recovering fully or that would predispose her to complications. Conditions that generally make patients ineligible for transplant include severe peripheral artery disease or cerebrovascular disease (strokes and aneurysms), irreversible dysfunction of another organ, cancer, irreversible pulmonary hypertension, and active systemic infection such as HIV/AIDS or tuberculosis that has spread throughout the body. In addition, candidates must be willing and able to comply with a complex medication schedule for the rest of their lives and are evaluated by a social worker or mental health professional.

In the United States, transplant candidates are placed on a waiting list maintained by the Organ Procurement and Transplantation Network/United Network for Organ Sharing (OPTN/UNOS). Allocation of hearts is based primarily on the severity of illness, time spent on the waiting list, blood type, body size, and geographic location of the donor organ. Guidelines prefer cardiac donors younger than fifty-five years with no history of chest trauma or heart disease, particularly coronary artery disease. Typically, multiple organs are procured from the donor at once, with several transplant teams present to focus on retrieving the heart, lungs, liver, and/or kidneys. After the heart is stopped and removed from the donor, it is inspected to make sure it is suitable for transplantation and packed in ice for transport. The heart can be kept on ice for a maximum of four to six hours.

The heart transplant operation is performed under general anesthesia. There are two types of procedures. The *orthotopic procedure*, in which the patient's heart is completely removed and replaced, is more commonly performed (see figure 7.3). In this procedure, the patient is put on the heart-lung machine, and his heart is stopped and removed. The new donor heart is sewn into place and then restarted, and the patient is weaned from the heart-lung machine. With the *heterotopic procedure*, the patient's own heart is left inside the body, and the donor heart is connected to it (see figure 7.4). This procedure may allow the patient's own heart the chance to recover. It is only performed in cases where the donor heart is not strong enough to function by itself.

If there are no complications following the operation, the patient will generally stay in the hospital for one to two weeks. Participation in a cardiac rehabilitation program may be recommended (see chapter 5), and the patient will be closely monitored for about three months at the heart transplant center. The monitoring may include frequent blood tests, lung function tests, ECGs, and echocardiograms (see chapter 3). Biopsies of heart tissue will also be obtained using cardiac catheterization in order to make sure that the body is not rejecting the new heart.

Rejection of the transplanted heart is a major concern, as the body's immune system attacks and destroys anything it perceives to be a foreign object. To prevent this, powerful immunosuppressive drugs are administered during the transplant operation and must be taken for the rest of the patient's life, in addition to a variety of other medications. The immunosuppressive drugs can cause many complications and are potentially toxic to the kidneys, so dosages must be closely monitored. Suppression of the immune system will also make the patient more susceptible to infections and to blood and skin cancers. During the first year following heart transplant, the risk is greatest that patients will die of infections or acute rejection of the heart or need to be hospitalized.

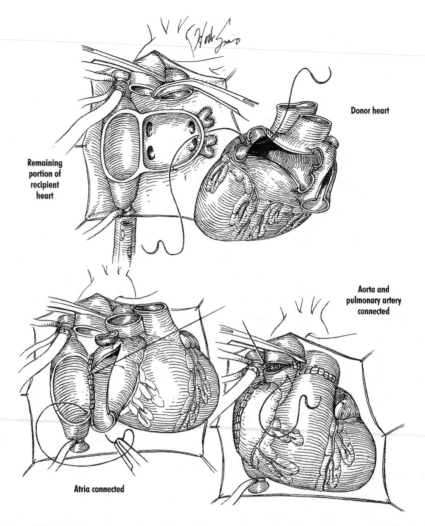

Donor heart

Remaining
portion of
recipient
heart

Aorta and
pulmonary artery
connected

Atria connected

Figure 7.3. Technique for orthotopic cardiac transplantation. *Illustration created by Herbert R. Smith Jr.*

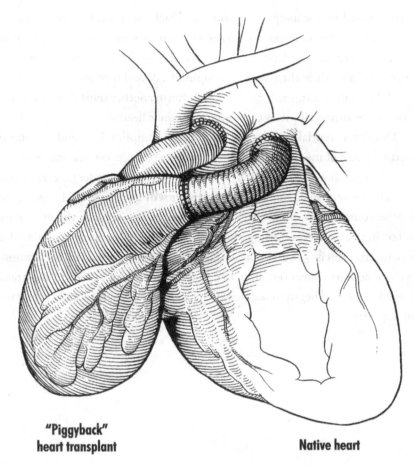

"Piggyback" heart transplant   **Native heart**

Figure 7.4. Technique for heterotopic or "piggyback" cardiac transplantation. *Illustration created by Herbert R. Smith Jr.*

About one-half of patients develop greatly accelerated, premature athero-sclerosis in the coronary arteries of the transplanted heart, sometimes referred to as *cardiac allograft vasculopathy* (CAV) or as *graft coronary artery disease*. This condition is a form of chronic, rather than acute, rejection of the donor heart and is the major factor preventing long-term survival in transplant patients. As with conventional forms of coronary artery disease, CAV can lead to heart attack, heart failure, and sudden death. Furthermore, when a patient receives a new heart, all of the nerves connected to the original heart are severed and not reattached. Thus, most patients are incapable of feeling chest pain, including angina caused by coronary artery disease, which can complicate diagnosis of this condition. Periodic cardiac catheterization may be required to check for coronary artery disease. Studies suggest that the use of statins following heart transplant can reduce the risk of developing CAV and increase chances of survival.[8] The only treatment for CAV is to perform another transplant operation, which is controversial given the scarcity of donor hearts.

Despite potential short- and long-term complications and a complicated schedule of medications, most transplant patients can resume relatively normal lives following surgery. Everyday activities and moderate exercise can generally be performed, although the patient will have a reduced capacity for exercise compared to individuals without heart disease. Since the new hearts do not have any nerves feeding them, they are not adequately stimulated in response to exercise, and the heart rate cannot properly adjust to changing levels of activity. However, after five years, regrowth of nerves to the transplanted heart may begin to occur, which can improve heart function and exercise capacity.

CHAPTER 8
VALVULAR HEART DISEASE

Four valves separate the chambers of the heart and keep blood flowing in a forward direction. These valves consist of leaflets arranged around circular openings that connect the different chambers of the heart. The valves operate of their own accord, without nerves or muscles to activate them. When the heart contracts, they respond to changes in pressure and open, allowing blood to flow through. Once blood passes from one chamber to the next, backward pressure from the moving blood causes the valve leaflets to close shut. Valvular heart disease occurs when these valves become damaged or deformed, either due to a birth defect or to acquired heart disease, and interfere with the normal pattern of blood flow. Valvular heart disease can also result if the shape of the heart changes due to aging or disease, thereby disturbing the natural alignment of the valve leaflets and hindering their normal function. These disruptions in flow cause the heart to work harder to keep the blood in circulation, and the heart may begin to enlarge. If left untreated, valvular disease can lead to heart failure over time.

Valvular heart disease has a variety of potential causes, ranging from birth defects to rare genetic disorders to the natural process of aging. This chapter focuses on the more common forms of valvular disease that typically arise later in life, rather than those caused by congenital or rare conditions. Many people with slightly abnormal valves may never experience symptoms and may require no treatment. In others, faulty valves can place limitations on physical activity due to symptoms of developing heart failure. Once a patient with valvular disease begins experiencing symptoms, surgical repair or replacement of the valve may be necessary. This chapter describes causes and characteristics of different types of valvular disease, as well as the latest advances in treatment.[1]

CAUSES AND CHARACTERISTICS

In the normally functioning heart, each of the four valves opens and closes at different points in the heartbeat. Initially, blood flows into the atria, or upper chambers of the heart, and the valves separating the atria from the ventricles, or lower chambers of the heart, are closed. When the atria contract, the pressure forces these valves open, and blood flows into the ventricles. The valve separating the atrium and ventricle on the right side of the heart is called the *tricuspid valve*, while the valve on the left is the *mitral valve* (see figures 6.1b and 6.2 in chapter 6). As the ventricles fill with blood and the pressure within them rises, the tricuspid and mitral valves close, and the first sound in the normal heartbeat is heard ("lub-DUB") (see figure 8.1). Next, the ventricles contract. On the right side of the heart, blood forces open the *pulmonary valve* as it enters the pulmonary artery to travel to the lungs. On the left side of the heart, blood passes through the *aortic valve* into the aorta, the major artery that supplies blood to the rest of the body. The second sound in the heartbeat is heard when the valves separating the ventricles from the pulmonary artery and the aorta close.

Valvular heart disease occurs when one or more valves, typically the mitral valve or the aortic valve on the left side of the heart, fail to function properly. The left side of the heart is responsible for receiving oxygen-rich blood and pumping it to the rest of the body, and dysfunction of the left ventricle puts a patient at high risk for heart failure (see chapter 7). Diseases of the tricuspid and pulmonary valves on the right side of the heart are much less common. Valvular disease takes two general forms. Either the opening through the valves becomes too narrow in a process called *stenosis* (the same term is used to describe the narrowing of arteries), or the valves fail to fully close, allowing blood to flow backward in a process called *regurgitation*. The term *insufficiency* may also be used to describe a leaky valve that fails to close. In many cases, a combination of stenosis and regurgitation is responsible for a faulty valve.

Valvular heart disease produces a *heart murmur*, which is an abnormal or extra sound heard during the heartbeat. It is generally first detected with a stethoscope during a routine physical examination, and it is often confirmed and further evaluated with an echocardiogram (see chapter 3). A heart murmur can indicate that one or more valves may be disrupting the flow of blood through the heart, although many murmurs are harmless and are not an indication of heart disease (functional murmurs). Some people will have a heart murmur that indicates a valvular abnormality, but they may never experience any other symptoms of valvular disease and require no further treatment. Others may have a heart murmur that is identified in childhood, and they may begin to develop symptoms only in middle age.

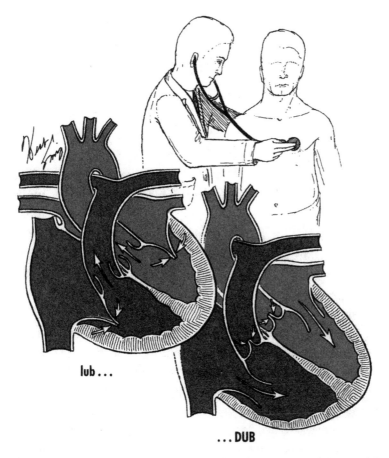

lub . . .

. . . DUB

Figure 8.1. The sounds in the heartbeat are caused by the opening and closing of the various valves of the heart. *Illustration created by Herbert R. Smith Jr.*

Symptoms of valvular disease vary depending on the valve affected; whether it is leaking, stenotic, or both; and the severity of the abnormality. Symptoms can include tiredness and fatigue, shortness of breath (dyspnea), and swelling in the lower body (edema) and can be similar to heart failure symptoms. Fatigue and weakness, commonly brought on by physical exertion, may occur because the skeletal muscles are not receiving a sufficient supply of blood and oxygen. Shortness of breath and swelling may develop if the normal flow of blood through the heart is impeded by narrowed or leaky valves. When this occurs, blood gets backed up, and fluid begins to leak into the lungs and other body tissues. In addition, the heart begins to enlarge as it works harder to pump blood. This enlargement of the heart, and particularly of the left ventricle, can worsen symptoms of heart failure.

Valvular disease can have a variety of causes. In the past, rheumatic fever was a major one. Rheumatic fever typically develops in children following untreated streptococcal throat infection or scarlet fever, and it causes inflammation throughout the body, particularly in the heart. The heart valves can become scarred and permanently damaged as a result. In the United States and other industrialized nations, rheumatic fever has become much less common since the development and widespread use of antibiotics, although it continues to be a problem in poor communities and developing countries. Some forms of valvular disease that are most often caused by rheumatic fever, such as *mitral stenosis*, have accordingly become less prevalent in the United States. However, other forms, such as *aortic stenosis*, which is associated with aging and may develop in a manner similar to atherosclerosis, have become more common as the population ages.

Heart attacks can damage the muscles or chords that anchor the heart valves, thereby interfering with their function. Due to the natural process of aging, the heart tissues supporting the valves can weaken or stretch, which can cause them to leak. Aging can also cause valves to become stiff, as calcium deposits begin to accumulate on them. Rarely, the valves and the inner surface of the heart can become infected with bacteria, resulting in *infective endocarditis*. This condition can be both a cause and a complication of valvular disease, as bacteria tend to become lodged on abnormal heart valves, causing further disease. Intravenous drug users are at higher risk of developing infective endocarditis by accidentally injecting bacteria into the bloodstream. Finally, a number of other conditions, including diseases and defects present at birth, can occasionally cause valvular disease. Examples include systemic lupus erythmatosis, carcinoid syndrome, metabolic disorders, and connective tissue disorders such as Marfan syndrome.

In the 1990s, a popular weight-loss drug, called Fen-Phen, and a related drug, dexfenfluramine (Redux), were found to cause valvular disease and *pulmonary hypertension*, or high blood pressure in the arteries supplying the lungs. These drugs produced *aortic insufficiency*, and sometimes *mitral insufficiency*, in susceptible patients, who in some cases had to undergo valve repair or replacement surgery. These drugs were taken off the market in 1997, although phentermine, one of the components of Fen-Phen not associated with valvular heart disease or pulmonary hypertension, remains available.

TYPES OF VALVULAR DISEASE

While any of the four heart valves can become dysfunctional, the aortic and mitral valves on the left side of the heart are the most often afflicted (see figures 8.2 and 8.3). Some patients may suffer from *multivalvular disease* affecting more than one valve.

Mitral stenosis is most often the result of rheumatic fever, although birth defects and a number of rare conditions are also potential causes. It is more common in women and may first be detected during pregnancy. It is characterized by a progressive thickening and stiffening of the valve leaflets, which may become fused together, resulting in a narrowing of the valve opening between the left atrium and ventricle. In addition, the tendons that anchor the mitral valve may thicken and contract. As the mitral valve opening becomes increasingly blocked, a murmur is produced during diastole (when the heart fills with blood). Blood flow from the left atrium to the ventricle is reduced, and pressure begins to build up in the atrium. This increase in pressure is transferred to the arteries and veins supplying the lungs, which results in pulmonary hypertension and fluid accumulation in the lungs, or pulmonary edema. The right ventricle is forced to work harder in order to pump blood

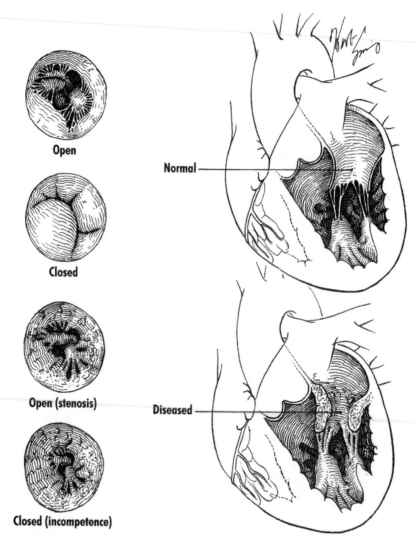

Figure 8.2. Mitral valve disease. *Illustration created by Herbert R. Smith Jr.*

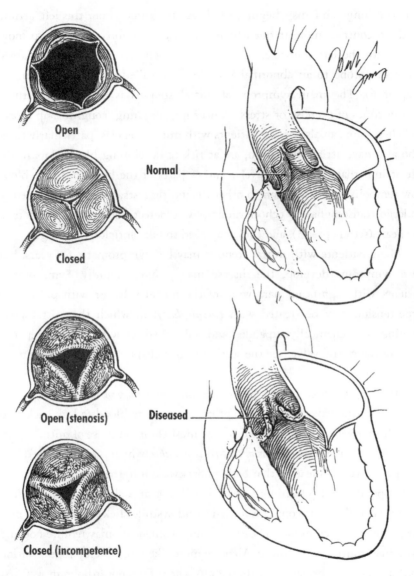

Figure 8.3. Aortic valve disease. *Illustration created by Herbert R. Smith Jr.*

into the lungs and may begin to fail. At the same time, the left atrium needs to contract more frequently and with greater force in order to move blood into the left ventricle. As a result, the left atrium becomes enlarged and more prone to an abnormal heart rhythm called atrial fibrillation (see chapter 6). The main symptom of mitral stenosis is difficulty breathing during times of exercise or stress. Wheezing, coughing, coughing up blood, and chest pain can also occur. Patients with mitral stenosis, particularly those who also have atrial fibrillation, are at risk of developing blood clots in the left atrium that may then travel to other parts of the body and stop blood flow (embolism). In addition to other diagnostic tests, patients may need to undergo transesophageal echocardiography to detect potential blood clots in the heart (see chapter 3), and they may need to take anticlotting drugs.

Many patients with mitral stenosis may be asymptomatic for years, but once symptoms develop, the disease may progress rapidly. Symptomatic patients with significant narrowing of the mitral valve or with pulmonary hypertension may be treated with *valvuloplasty*, in which the mitral valve opening is mechanically expanded and unblocked, or with surgical replacement of the mitral valve (see the section in this chapter on valve replacement and repair).

Mitral regurgitation, also known as *mitral insufficiency* or *incompetence*, occurs when the mitral valve fails to close properly, allowing blood to leak backward from the left ventricle to the atrium. The most common cause of mitral regurgitation in the United States is *mitral valve prolapse*, which is characterized by a "floppy" valve with leaflets that balloon backward into the atrium like a parachute opening. The examining physician may hear a clicking sound during systole when the heart contracts (called a mid-systolic click). Mitral valve prolapse is relatively common in healthy, young women and may require nothing other than routine monitoring. Men are more likely to develop regurgitation from mitral valve prolapse. In the 1980s, when the echocardiogram was first introduced, mitral valve prolapse was overly diagnosed, and the condition was believed to affect as much as 15 percent of the population. Now, as standards regarding echocardiography have become more uniform, it appears that mitral valve prolapse is present in less than 3 percent of individuals. In many individuals, mitral valve prolapse is a benign condition associated with no symptoms, but in others, mitral insufficiency and arrhythmias can develop. Other potential causes of mitral regurgitation include rheumatic fever and infective endocarditis, which can damage the valve leaflets, and cardiomyopathy, or enlargement of the heart, which can cause the ring of tissue surrounding the valve to expand. Calcium deposits can also form on this surrounding ring of tissue, in a process similar to atherosclerosis, and prevent the valves from fully closing. In addition, the tendons that anchor the mitral valve may tear, or the *papillary muscles* attached to these tendons may become scarred or deformed by a heart attack.

With mitral regurgitation, the left ventricle is forced to pump larger amounts of blood with each contraction and gradually increases in size. The backward flow of blood also increases pressure in the left atrium, which causes fluid to leak back into the lungs, and a murmur is heard during systole (contraction) over the heart and radiating to the left armpit. Atrial fibrillation may develop. Symptoms include shortness of breath, fatigue, and swelling. Patients may remain asymptomatic for many years, and mitral regurgitation does not generally become rapidly severe unless infective endocarditis develops or the tendons anchoring the mitral valve tear. Surgery is recommended for patients who have symptoms of heart failure or who are asymptomatic but are showing signs of developing left ventricular dysfunction or enlargement. Reconstructing the mitral valve surgically to restore its normal function is generally considered preferable to replacement, except in older adults who have severely damaged valves.

Aortic stenosis refers to the narrowing of the opening through which blood flows from the heart to the aorta and on to the rest of the body. It can be caused by a birth defect or rheumatic fever or, more commonly, acquired in a manner similar to atherosclerosis. In this latter form, calcium deposits develop on the valve leaflets, causing them to thicken and eventually become incapable of movement. Previously, aortic stenosis was believed to be solely a result of aging, but it now appears that risk factors for atherosclerosis, including high cholesterol, diabetes, smoking, and hypertension, also predispose individuals to aortic stenosis. People with aortic stenosis are at higher risk for heart attack, and recently researchers investigated the possibility that lipid-lowering drugs such as statins might be beneficial for the prevention and treatment of aortic stenosis.[2] Statin therapy did not slow the progression of aortic stenosis or reduce the need for valve replacement, although the two conditions share risk factors and other similarities. Statins are not currently recommended for the prevention or treatment of aortic stenosis.

Aortic stenosis impedes the flow of blood from the left ventricle, which causes the heart to work harder and the left ventricle to enlarge. A murmur is heard during systole (contraction) radiating to the neck. Patients may experience no symptoms as the disease progresses, but ultimately, symptoms of heart failure develop, with attacks of shortness of breath, chest pain, and loss of consciousness. Aortic stenosis may mimic or worsen the symptoms of coronary artery disease, particularly the chest pain of angina (see chapter 4). Patients with severe aortic stenosis may experience gastrointestinal bleeding. By the time symptoms develop, aortic stenosis is often severe, and replacement of the aortic valve may be required within a short period of time. Without surgical treatment, patients may live only one to three years after developing symptoms.

Aortic regurgitation, also referred to as *aortic insufficiency* or *incompetence*, can result from rheumatic fever or infective endocarditis, which may directly damage the aortic valve itself. More commonly, diseases and conditions that weaken or enlarge the *aortic root*, or the part of the aorta attached to the heart, cause the aortic valve to leak. These potential causes include stretching of the aortic root due to aging, tears or dissections of the aorta, various forms of inflammatory disorders including inflammatory arthritis, connective tissue disorders such as Marfan syndrome, and high blood pressure. Before the advent of antibiotics, advanced syphilis was a relatively common cause of aortic regurgitation. With aortic regurgitation, blood pumped out of the left ventricle partially leaks back, which increases the workload on the heart and causes it to enlarge and ultimately fail. As with aortic stenosis, patients may not experience symptoms for a number of years, but, once they do, aortic regurgitation progresses rapidly and generally requires valve replacement. Symptoms include shortness of breath during exercise, while lying down, and while asleep; fatigue; chest pain, including at night; and an uncomfortable pounding of the heart or head. Physical examination may reveal a diastolic murmur (while the heart fills with blood) and what is known as a "water-hammer pulse." Surgery is recommended for all patients with symptoms who are able to undergo surgery, as well as for asymptomatic patients who are showing signs of developing failure of the left ventricle. In some patients who have aortic regurgitation because of an enlarged aortic root, this area can be surgically tightened without the need for valve replacement. In other patients, including those with combined aortic stenosis and regurgitation, the aortic valve will need to be replaced.

Diseases of the tricuspid and pulmonary valves are much less common. *Tricuspid stenosis* is almost always caused by rheumatic fever and frequently occurs along with tricuspid regurgitation, mitral stenosis, or aortic stenosis. Repair or replacement of the tricuspid valve generally occurs in conjunction with procedures to correct other diseased valves. *Tricuspid regurgitation* is most often a complication of failure of the right ventricle, and patients also frequently have mitral valve disease. Tricuspid regurgitation does not usually require treatment. *Pulmonic stenosis* is generally due to birth defects. *Pulmonic regurgitation* is most often a complication of pulmonary hypertension, but it rarely requires treatment.

DIAGNOSIS AND MEDICAL TREATMENT

For many individuals, detection of a heart murmur with a stethoscope during a routine examination may provide the first indication of potential valvular disease. Each of the different forms of valvular disease produces a characteristic sound caused by abnormal blood flow through the heart. A physician may also be able to identify valvular disease by feeling the pulse at different points throughout the body. If a heart murmur or abnormal pulse is detected, echocardiography is typically employed to confirm a diagnosis (see chapter 3). Echocardiography provides a moving picture of the heart using ultrasound, and it allows doctors to evaluate the structure and movement of the valves, identify the presence of calcium deposits, and measure the speed of blood flow through the chambers. Transesophageal echocardiography may be used to look for blood clots in the left atrium or to obtain more detailed images than are possible with standard transthoracic echocardiography. Sometimes exercise testing will be combined with echocardiography to determine how well the heart functions during times of physical stress. Echocardiograms, x-rays, and electrocardiography can also indicate if the heart is enlarged, and electrocardiography can show whether an abnormal heart rhythm is developing in conjunction with valvular disease.

Echocardiography is generally the primary means of diagnosing and eval-uating valvular disease, but on occasion, additional images may be needed. Nuclear imaging, magnetic resonance imaging (MRI), and computed tomog-raphy (CT) can sometimes provide further information about the size and function of the heart. Cardiac catheterization may be performed if there is doubt surrounding a diagnosis of valvular disease or if the patient is also suspected of having coronary artery disease. (The authors once examined an elderly patient who was experiencing chest discomfort and shortness of breath with physical exertion and who had an exceptionally loud murmur of aortic stenosis. On cardiac catheterization, the patient was found to have no sig-nificant pressure gradient across the aortic valve, which eliminated the need to replace the valve, but coronary angiography showed that there was severe triple-vessel coronary artery disease.) In addition to identifying blockages within the arteries, cardiac catheterization can be used to measure pressures within different chambers of the heart.

Patients with valvular disease who do not have symptoms often do not require any treatment. Depending on the severity of their underlying condi-tions and the risk of developing future heart failure, they may be asked to schedule regular follow-up visits to the doctor so that heart size and function can be periodically monitored with echocardiography. These visits may range in frequency from every six months to every five years. Patients should inform their doctors immediately if symptoms of heart failure begin to develop.

There are no drugs specifically for valvular disease, and currently the only way to treat a faulty valve is to repair or replace it. Drugs to alleviate symptoms of heart failure may be prescribed to delay the need for valvular surgery or to treat patients who are not candidates for surgery. These drugs may include diuretics to reduce swelling and fluid accumulation, as well as ACE inhibitors or vasodilators to reduce blood pressure and improve blood flow. Patients who develop abnormal heart rhythms such as atrial fibrillation may need to take drugs for these conditions. These patients may also need to take anticlotting drugs to prevent embolism, as the formation of clots in the heart that subsequently travel through the bloodstream is more common in patients with both valvular heart disease and atrial fibrillation.

For many decades, the American Heart Association has recommended that people with valvular disease routinely take antibiotics before certain dental and surgical procedures in order to prevent the development of infective endocarditis. This recommendation was based on the assumption that a common cause of infective endocarditis is bacteria typically found in the mouth and that some procedures could release this bacteria into the bloodstream. In 2007, the AHA revised its policy and no longer recommends antibiotic use before many surgical procedures.[3] In addition, only people with prosthetic (artificial) heart valves, previous history of endocarditis, heart transplant with abnormal valvular function, or certain congenital heart defects are advised to take antibiotics before dental procedures. It is now believed that the number of infections prevented with routine antibiotic use is very small and that the best way to guard against infective endocarditis is by maintaining good oral health.

VALVE REPLACEMENT AND REPAIR

Many patients who develop symptoms of valvular disease will need to have the malfunctioning valve(s) repaired or replaced. Traditionally, the only way to fix a damaged heart valve has been through open-heart surgery. These procedures require a high level of surgical skill, but refinements in techniques and advances in the construction of prosthetic valves have made surgery an increasingly common treatment option. In the early 1980s, it first became possible to repair valves using cardiac catheterization. This kind of *percutaneous* approach, which is even more technically demanding than surgical valve repair or replacement, can be successfully employed in limited cases. In general, long-term outcomes with percutaneous valve repair and replacement have been mixed. Researchers continue to work on developing minimally invasive procedures for the treatment of valvular disease. These experimental techniques are likely to benefit a large number of people since many patients with valvular disease are elderly and have other health conditions that make open-heart surgery too risky an option. Advanced age increases the risks associated with open-heart surgery, but many elderly patients still gain considerable benefit.

Doctors often need to decide whether candidates for surgery should undergo valve repair or valve replacement. Most people with a faulty aortic valve who have surgery will undergo valve replacement, which has better long-term results than aortic valve repair. In contrast, repair of the mitral valve is considered preferable to replacement because of the risks associated with *prosthetic valves*. Prosthetic valves can be either mechanical heart valves that are made out of metal and synthetic materials or tissue valves (also called bioprosthetic valves) that are made often using tissue from animals, most commonly pigs and cows (see figure 8.4). Tissue valves can additionally be obtained from human cadavers or constructed from a patient's own pericardium (membrane surrounding the heart). The risk of blood clot formation is higher with mechanical valves, so patients are required to take anticlotting drugs and aspirin for the rest of their lives. Tissue valves require anticlotting drugs only for the first three months after implantation, but they tend to deteriorate, in some patients as soon as five years following valve replacement. Bioprosthetic valves break down more quickly in patients younger than thirty-five years of age and are not recommended in this population. Both mechanical and tissue valves also increase risk for infective endocarditis; therefore, patients with prosthetic valves are advised to take antibiotics before dental procedures.

Mitral Valve

Patients with mitral stenosis can sometimes be treated with valvuloplasty or *valvotomy*, a procedure that widens the blocked valvular opening. *Balloon valvotomy* is a percutaneous technique similar to the one used to unblock clogged arteries. It is performed with the patient mildly sedated. One or two balloon catheters are inserted through the femoral artery in the groin or through a small puncture in the chest, and they are guided into the heart. The balloons are then expanded to separate valve leaflets that may have become fused together or coated with calcium deposits. The procedure is especially successful in younger patients without severely damaged valves, and it results in improved symptoms and reduced pressure in the lungs. The risk of complications, including clot formation, puncture of the heart, and mitral regurgitation, is low. Valvotomy can also be performed as open-heart surgery in patients with more deformed valves. With both balloon valvotomy and surgical valvotomy, restenosis, or reclosing, of the mitral valve, in addition to regurgitation, may occur and may possibly require future valve replacement. However, patients generally remain free of symptoms for ten to fifteen years following the initial procedure.

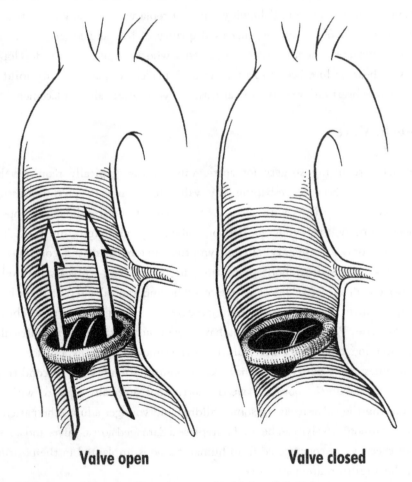

Valve open   **Valve closed**

Figure 8.4. A prosthetic valve. *Illustration created by Herbert R. Smith Jr.*

In many patients with mitral regurgitation, the valve can be surgically repaired. Repair involves reshaping the valve and the surrounding tissue to restore normal function, as well as sometimes implanting a prosthetic ring around the valve for support. Patients with severe mitral stenosis or mitral regurgitation who are older and have very stiff and deformed valves may need to have their valves replaced. Mitral valve repair and replacement are open-heart procedures performed with the patient under general anesthesia. The risk of surgery is increased in patients who are undergoing simultaneous coronary artery bypass graft (CABG) surgery (see chapter 5) or who have severe left ventricular dysfunction. Following repair or replacement, many patients have improvement of symptoms, increased quality of life, and longer life spans. Outcomes are generally better in patients who have not already developed severe heart failure before surgery, with 75 percent of patients with mild to moderate heart failure surviving at least ten years after valve replacement.

Aortic Valve

Patients requiring surgery for aortic valve disease typically require valve replacement because reshaping the valve tends not to produce lasting results. Some patients with aortic stenosis who are not candidates for open-heart surgery may undergo balloon valvotomy, although this procedure provides only a temporary relief of symptoms before the disease continues to progress. Approximately 85 percent of patients are alive ten years after valve replacement surgery. Almost all patients who undergo valve replacement have improvement of symptoms, including reduced chest pain and increased ability to exercise. Patients who do not have severe heart failure, left ventricular dysfunction, or coronary artery disease at the time of surgery experience better outcomes. Some patients who have aortic regurgitation because of conditions affecting the aortic root can have the aortic root surgically repaired without replacing the valve itself. In some children and younger adults, the patient's own pulmonary valve can be used to replace a damaged aortic valve, and a new prosthetic valve constructed from human tissue is implanted in the position of the original pulmonary valve.

Tricuspid and Pulmonic Valves

Diseases of the tricuspid and pulmonary valves are rarely severe enough to require valve repair or replacement. If necessary, the valves can be repaired percutaneously by valvuloplasty, but sometimes open-heart surgery to repair or replace faulty valves is warranted.

Minimally Invasive Valve Repair and Replacement

Percutaneous balloon valvotomy, or valvuloplasty, is one minimally invasive procedure that can sometimes be employed to widen blocked heart valves. It is most successful in treating mitral and pulmonic stenosis; it is less commonly used for patients with aortic stenosis. In recent decades, doctors have experimented with other procedures that would allow them to repair or replace damaged valves without performing open-heart surgery, in which the breastbone is divided through an incision down the middle of the chest. Surgeries involving smaller incisions in the chest, for example, could speed recovery, reduce the risk for infection, and be particularly useful in patients who have already undergone heart surgery. Another variation is *port-access surgery*, in which surgical instruments are inserted through small incisions in the chest and the procedure is viewed on a video monitor. In theory, robots could help facilitate these technically difficult procedures. In general, however, minimally invasive surgical procedures for valve repair and replacement are still considered experimental, as long-term results have not been as good as those produced by traditional surgery.

Percutaneous approaches to valve repair and replacement are currently being tested. Recent attempts to replace aortic valves with the use of catheters instead of surgery, referred to as *transcatheter aortic valve implantation*, have been promising.[4] A few companies in the United States have developed metal valves that can be inserted through the femoral artery in the groin and directed into the heart; alternatively, these valves can be inserted through a small incision in the chest, between the ribs. Once the valve is in position, it is expanded and begins to take over the function of the damaged valve. A percutaneous approach to mitral valve repair is also under investigation in patients with mitral valve regurgitation.[5] In this procedure, a small, metal clip is delivered through a catheter inserted into the femoral artery in the groin and then directed to the heart. The clip is attached to the flaps of the mitral valve to hold them in place and prevent leakage, and the catheter is withdrawn. Frail, elderly patients who are not considered candidates for open-heart surgery may be the most likely to benefit from these kinds of advanced technology, at least initially. While currently available in Europe, these new valves are now being tested in the United States in older patients not eligible for surgery. As researchers learn more about how the valves perform, their use might also extend to younger patients seeking a less traumatic alternative to open-heart surgery.

CHAPTER 9

THE FUTURE OF CARDIOVASCULAR MEDICINE

In recent decades, enormous progress has been made in the prevention, diagnosis, and treatment of cardiovascular disease. Doctors starting out today are able to do things to help their patients that were unimaginable just fifty years ago. As we have seen in the preceding chapters, medical imaging, drug therapies, surgical and minimally invasive techniques, and implantable devices have all advanced to high levels of sophistication, resulting in increased longevity and improved quality of life for millions of people. Now, in the twenty-first century, we have gained great insights into how heart disease develops and how to prevent and treat it if necessary.

Still, some of the most exciting advances in cardiology may be yet to come. The sequencing of the human genome, first completed in 2003, was a major breakthrough in medical science. It yielded a wealth of information that scientists are just beginning to interpret fully. We now know the sequence and location of the approximately twenty-five thousand genes in the human genome. Thirty years ago, we had information on a fraction of this number, probably fewer than one hundred genes. The first human genome took more than one decade to sequence, at a cost of about three billion dollars, and it was a composite of the DNA from several individuals. Today, with the development of fast and inexpensive sequencers, it is possible to sequence one person's genome in about one week for just thousands of dollars.

The sequencing of the human genome is allowing researchers to determine how the genetic makeup of humans differs from that of other organisms, and it is also providing information on how different human beings are from each other. While much of the human genome is the same from one person to

247

the next, scientists have found that the genomes of different individuals vary in approximately 1 to 3 percent of the sequence.[1] In its entirety, the human genome is about three billion base pairs long. (DNA consists of two strands of nucleotides arranged in a double helix. Each nucleotide has one of four different bases. A base pair refers to two nucleotides on opposite strands that hold the strands together via hydrogen bonds.) Thus, each person's genome contains about four million sequences that are different from others in the general population. About three million of these variations are *single-nucleotide polymorphisms* (SNPs, pronounced "snips"), or substitutions of just one base. These kinds of *genetic variants*, which can be as simple as having one base as opposed to another in a gene sequence composed of thousands of bases, can theoretically have wide-ranging effects. Genes code for proteins, and a substitution of one base could potentially change the shape of a protein, which could alter its function. This alteration could subsequently affect a particular individual's susceptibility to a disease or change how he responds to a drug, vaccine, or other type of stimulus. The majority of genetic variants do not have any apparent effect on human health, however, and many diseases are influenced by multiple genes, as well as by factors such as environment and lifestyle.

A new model within medical science is *translational research*, which aims to speed the transition between laboratory research and patient care. The goal is to conduct research that will quickly lead to improved treatments and better medical technologies. With the sequencing of the human genome, researchers are now amassing data on genetic factors that may affect the development of heart disease. As research in this field continues to accumulate, scientists are coming ever closer to making *personalized medicine* a reality. Personalized medicine would incorporate information about an individual's genetic makeup into all stages of medical care, including prevention, diagnosis, and treatment. *Gene therapy* and *stem cell therapy* also have the potential to transform cardiovascular medicine, possibly by helping to regenerate damaged heart tissue.

PERSONALIZED MEDICINE

Since the 1970s, many new scientific fields have emerged as our technological capabilities have expanded. For example, *genomics* is the study of all of the genes in a cell or in an organism, while *proteomics* is the study of all of the proteins. An individual's genes remain constant throughout a lifetime, but different genes are expressed as proteins by different cells at different times. Thus, levels of proteins in a cell or in an organism are constantly changing. Genomics and proteomics, in addition to other emerging scientific fields, are contributing to the development of personalized medicine. The goal of personalized medicine is to understand how the vast amounts of information encoded by our genes and available through analysis of our proteins can lead to better strategies for prevention, diagnosis, and treatment. Personalized medicine is still in its infancy, although much progress has been made in the area of cancer diagnosis and treatment in particular.

In theory, personalized medicine could help identify individuals who are at increased risk for cardiovascular disease well before symptoms arise. Traditionally, cardiovascular disease prevention has relied on the management of risk factors, such as high cholesterol, high blood pressure, diabetes, and smoking. However, there are many individuals who develop heart disease despite having only one, or none, of the traditional risk factors. Researchers have been looking for new ways to screen for cardiovascular disease by trying to identify genes or proteins that may help predict whether a given individual is likely to be at increased risk.

Scientists have currently identified at least twenty-three areas within the genome, called genetic loci, that can be associated with increased risk for coronary artery disease, depending on whether an individual carries certain genetic variants.[2] Some of these genetic variants affect traditional cardiovascular risk factors, such as levels of LDL-C, HDL-C, and hypertension. For example, variations in the *PCSK9* gene can profoundly affect LDL-C levels. One type of *PCSK9* mutation results in extremely high LDL-C levels, similar to those found in individuals with a rare hereditary disorder called familial hypercholesterolemia. Another kind of *PCSK9* mutation results in lifelong low cholesterol levels, causing reductions in LDL-C of 28 percent in African Americans and of 15 percent in Caucasians.[3] Individuals with these genetic variants are at decreased risk for coronary heart disease: risk has been reported to be reduced by 88 percent in African Americans and by 47 percent in Caucasians.

Many of the other genetic loci associated with coronary artery disease do not appear to affect the traditional cardiovascular risk factors, and many are located on genes that were previously believed to be unrelated to the development of coronary artery disease. A region located on chromosome 9, referred to as chromosome 9p21, has been widely studied by investigators.[4] Approximately one-half of the population is believed to have one SNP at 9p21 that is associated with increased risk for cardiovascular disease, and about one-quarter have two SNPs. People with two of the variants are estimated as having a 25 percent greater risk for heart disease compared to people with only one, while people with none have a 25 percent lower risk for heart disease compared to people with only one. Yet the 9p21 chromosome is not associated with any known genes, which provides some indication of the complexity of genetic research. Genetic testing for 9p21 and other variants is still considered experimental and is not currently being used by physicians to screen for coronary artery disease.

While there are thousands of diseases that are caused by mutations in single genes, such as sickle cell anemia and cystic fibrosis, there are also more common diseases, including coronary heart disease, diabetes, and cancer, that are affected by multiple genes in combination with lifestyle and environmental factors. Having one or more SNPs associated with heart disease can increase cardiovascular risk; nonetheless, it appears that lifestyle still plays a large role in determining who will actually develop heart disease. One form that personalized medicine could take would be to help identify people who may be more susceptible to developing heart disease because of their genetics. These individuals would then receive tailored treatments to prevent heart disease, including intensified control of risk factors.

One goal of personalized medicine is to use genomic and proteomic research to improve diagnosis of cardiovascular disease. By analyzing gene expression and levels of proteins in both diseased and healthy heart tissue, researchers may be able to identify molecular patterns associated with different heart conditions. For example, patients with advanced heart failure may have different levels of proteins compared to those with mild heart failure or with healthy hearts. If researchers were able to identify these kinds of markers for advanced heart failure, diagnosis, which currently incorporates a patient's reporting of symptoms, would become more standardized and accurate. It would also allow doctors to better track a patient's disease across time and to determine the most effective course of treatment at each stage. Brain natriuretic peptide, which was discovered in 1988, is an example of a protein that is currently being used to help identify patients with heart failure; studies are currently investigating its potential relevance to other conditions. In the field of cancer research, scientists have been able to distinguish cancer cells from healthy cells based on their DNA content, instead of examining tissue biopsies under a microscope. They have also been able to identify patterns of genes that indicate which patients are likely to have a better prognosis and which are more likely to respond to standard treatments, and they are developing new screening tests for cancer based on different levels of proteins in the blood. While many of these approaches are still experimental in the field of cancer research, scientists are hopeful that similar techniques will be developed for the diagnosis and improved treatment of heart disease.

Personalized medicine is closer to becoming a reality as it pertains to treatment with cardiovascular drugs. Traditionally, physicians have used large studies, often enrolling thousands of people, to determine how to best treat patients with a particular disease. These kinds of studies, including those used to test new drugs, can indicate how people in general may tend to react to a treatment, what appears to be a good average dose, and what side effects are likely to emerge. However, they cannot predict how any given person will react to a specific medication. For one person, a drug may work as anticipated, while another might need a higher dose. Someone else might develop worrisome side effects if prescribed that particular drug and should instead be given something else. In some cases, these differences in response to medications are determined by genetic differences. Currently, doctors may choose to conduct genetic testing before prescribing more than seventy commonly used drugs.

Genetic tests exist for a few cardiovascular drugs. In 2007, the FDA approved genetic testing for the anticoagulant drug warfarin, which is used to prevent the formation of blood clots (see chapters 5 and 7 for more on warfarin).[5] According to the FDA, in about one-third of patients, warfarin is metabolized differently than expected, and its blood-thinning action carries an increased risk for serious internal bleeding. Doctors have traditionally estimated initial doses based on a patient's weight, age, and other factors. The FDA approved genetic testing for warfarin based on observations that variants of two genes, *CYP2C9* and *VKORC1*, can make patients more sensitive to warfarin. These patients would then require lower doses. In 2010, a nationwide study reported that people on warfarin who had undergone genetic testing were about 30 percent less likely to be hospitalized compared to people who had not.[6] Genetic testing for another anticlotting drug, the antiplatelet agent clopidogrel, was approved in 2010. According to the FDA, individuals with variants of the *CYP2C19* gene do not metabolize clopidogrel well, so it works less effectively and places them at increased risk for blood clotting leading to heart attack and other ischemic events.[7]

Genetic variants have also been identified that can affect an individual's response to statins and beta-blockers. For example, people with variants in the *SLCO1B1* gene have been found to be more susceptible to muscle-related side effects from statins, while individuals with SNPs in the *APOE* gene may have lesser reductions in LDL-C while on statin drugs compared to others.[8] Similarly, a variant in the *ADRB1* gene, which is commonly found in African Americans but is rare in whites, can make beta-blockers work less effectively in people with systolic heart failure.[9] Genetic testing before prescribing statins and beta-blockers is not currently conducted, and it may be some years before genetic testing for anticlotting agents becomes widespread in everyday clinical practice.

GENE THERAPY

Gene therapy is the process of introducing genetic material, in the form of DNA or RNA, into a cell in order to alter the pattern of gene expression in that cell. Sometimes a gene may be defective or missing, and the new genetic material is designed to help restore normal cell function. At other times, genetic material is introduced into a normally functioning cell in order to selectively increase or decrease levels of gene expression. Although the concept has been in existence at least since the 1970s, gene therapy approaches currently remain experimental within cardiovascular medicine.

Genes can be delivered into cells outside of the body by first removing them, genetically modifying them in a lab, and then returning the modified cells to the body. Or cells can be modified within the body by introducing genetic material through a vehicle referred to as a vector. In cardiovascular medicine, the vectors that have been used most successfully have been viruses. The viruses are modified so that they do not cause disease, and the new genetic information is inserted into them. The vectors containing genetic material can then be introduced into the body through injection into the bloodstream with the use of catheters or by direct injection into the heart or other tissues. The viruses subsequently infect cells at the target site and replicate their genetic material, and, ideally, levels of gene expression are altered.

The current focus of cardiovascular gene therapy research is the growth of new blood vessels in tissues damaged by atherosclerotic vascular disease.[10] As discussed in chapter 4, atherosclerotic disease can cause blood vessels to narrow or become completely blocked, leading to a deficiency in the normal supply of blood and oxygen that can permanently damage tissues and organs. Researchers have explored gene therapy to stimulate the growth of new blood vessels and restore blood flow in patients who are unable to be treated by conventional approaches, including drugs, bypass surgery, or percutaneous intervention. The strategy is to introduce genetic material to increase expression of specialized proteins that cause cells to grow and differentiate into new blood vessels. Other studies have explored gene therapy for the prevention of restenosis, or the reclosing of a blood vessel after it has been unblocked with a stent or bypass surgery (see chapter 5). Research has also examined potential treatments for heart failure that would work by increasing the strength of the contractions of heart cells and by preventing the heart from enlarging and changing shape.

In general, gene therapy faces some obstacles before becoming widely used. Scientists are still trying to determine the optimal way to deliver genetic material into cells so that the desired effects last long enough and occur at appropriate levels. Many of the viruses used as vectors only alter gene expression for a few weeks at a time and can sometimes cause inflammatory reactions as side effects. Yet gene therapy remains a promising area of investigation within cardiovascular medicine, and researchers are optimistic that advances in this field will lead to improved treatments for heart disease.

STEM CELL THERAPY

Stem cell research is one of the most exciting fields in science today. It holds out the possibility that physicians may one day be able to repair or replace damaged cells, tissues, and organs on a molecular level. Of course, stem cell research is also surrounded by controversy, particularly regarding the use of embryonic stem cells. However, scientists have discovered many new sources of stem cells, which has helped address some of these concerns. As stem cell research continues to advance, it is becoming increasingly likely that innovative therapies for diseases such as heart disease, Alzheimer's, Parkinson's, stroke, diabetes, and cancer will be developed. Stem cell therapy has already been used since 1968 in bone marrow transplants to treat individuals with leukemia and related cancers.

What makes stem cells so potentially powerful within the world of medicine is their ability to self-replicate and differentiate into many different kinds of cells. Embryonic stem cells are *pluripotent*, which means that they are capable of differentiating into any of the more than two hundred types of cells found in an adult human, given the proper stimuli and conditions. The majority of adult stem cells are not pluripotent, although some pluripotent adult stem cells can be found in places such as umbilical cord blood. Most adult stem cells are capable of differentiating only into a closely related family of cells. For example, a blood stem cell can differentiate into a number of different types of blood cell, but not into a heart or nerve cell.

A major advance within the past several years has been the successful reprogramming of regular adult body cells into pluripotent stem cells. These *induced pluripotent cells* are created by using specialized proteins to trigger the expression of specific genes within the adult body cell so that they resemble embryonic stem cells. The first induced pluripotent stem cells were created from mouse body cells in 2006 and from humans in 2007.[11] Many different kinds of human body cells, including cells derived from the skin, gums, hair, and testes, can be reprogrammed to become pluripotent. Theoretically, in the future, scientists may be able to create induced pluripotent stem cells to treat individual patients with stem cells derived from their own bodies. A hurdle currently facing researchers is the tendency of these kinds of cells to cause tumors.

Although many stem cell studies are still being conducted in animal models or in laboratory experiments, scientists hope to soon translate their findings to repair or regenerate damaged hearts in humans. Many survivors of heart attacks have areas of dead tissue, which can lead to heart failure. Heart failure from other causes is also associated with injury and death to heart cells. In adult humans, the heart muscle regenerates itself very slowly, and the number of heart cells that can be naturally replaced following injury from a heart attack or another form of heart disease is limited. The major strategy under investigation is the prevention and treatment of heart failure by introducing stem cells into the damaged heart in order to stimulate the growth of new contractile heart cells.[12] Stem cells could be delivered by injections into the bloodstream or directly into the heart, or delivered by catheters. As researchers gain an increased understanding of which kinds of stem cells are the most effective for cardiovascular therapy and how they should be delivered, we come closer to one day being able to repair damaged human hearts at a cellular level. Now is an exciting time in science and medicine, as we witness the development of technologies and therapies that would never before have been thought possible.

ACKNOWLEDGMENTS

Numerous colleagues have contributed their time and expertise to the prior editions of this book. Their efforts, particularly the illustrations by Herbert R. Smith Jr., continue to enrich the current version. We would like to thank John Farmer, MD, and Guillermo Torre-Amione, MD, in Houston, Texas, who provided invaluable feedback during the planning stages for this project. We greatly appreciate the assistance of George Bell, MD, who reviewed the chapters dealing with the diagnosis and management of different forms of heart disease. We are also grateful to Frank Weimann and Elyse Tanzillo at The Literary Group International and to Steven L. Mitchell, Linda Greenspan Regan, and everyone at Prometheus Books for bringing this project to fruition. Special thanks goes to Jennifer Moon, PhD, for her research and writing assistance with this book.

NOTES

PREFACE

1. Earl S. Ford et al., "Explaining the Decrease in U.S. Deaths from Coronary Disease, 1980–2000," *New England Journal of Medicine* 356, no. 23 (2007): 2388–98.

2. Véronique L. Roger et al., "Heart Disease and Stroke Statistics 2011 Update: A Report from the American Heart Association," *Circulation* 123, no. 4 (2011): e18–209.

3. Ford et al., "Explaining the Decrease in U.S. Deaths," pp. 2388–98.

CHAPTER 1. CHOLESTEROL AND ATHEROSCLEROSIS: THE NEW BIOLOGY

1. Véronique L. Roger et al., "Heart Disease and Stroke Statistics 2011 Update: A Report from the American Heart Association," *Circulation* 123, no. 4 (2011): e18–209.

2. Felix J. Marchand, "Über Arteriosklerose," in *Verhandlungen der Kongresse für Innere Medizin*, 21 Kongresse, ed. E. von Leyden and E. Pfeiffer (Wiesbaden, Ger.: Verlag von J.F. Bergmann, 1904), pp. 23–59.

3. Nikolai N. Anichkov, S. Chalatow, "Über experimentelle Cholesterinsteatose und ihre Bedeutung für die Entstehung einiger pathologischer Prozesse," *Zentralblatt für Allgemeine Pathologie* 24 (1913): 1–9.

4. W. M. Monique Verschuren et al., "Serum Total Cholesterol and Long-Term Coronary Heart Disease Mortality in Different Cultures. Twenty-Five-Year Follow-Up of the Seven Countries Study," *Journal of the American Medical Association* 274, no. 2 (1995): 131–36.

5. Thomas L. Robertson et al., "Epidemiologic Studies of Coronary Heart Disease and Stroke in Japanese Men Living in Japan, Hawaii and California. Incidence of Myocardial Infarction and Death from Coronary Heart Disease," *American Journal of Cardiology* 39, no. 2 (1977): 239–43.

6. William B. Kannel et al., "Factors of Risk in the Development of Coronary Heart Disease—Six Year Follow-Up Experience. The Framingham Study," *Annals of Internal Medicine* 55 (1961): 33–50.

7. JoAnn E. Manson et al., "The Primary Prevention of Myocardial Infarction," *New England Journal of Medicine* 326, no. 2 (1992): 1406–16.

8. Peter Libby, Paul M. Ridker, Göran K. Hansson, "Progress and Challenges in Translating the Biology of Atherosclerosis," *Nature* 473 (2011): 317–25.

9. Russell Ross, John Glomset, Laurence Harker, "Response to Injury and Atherogenesis," *American Journal of Pathology* 86 (1977): 675–84.

10. Kevin J. Williams, Ira Tabas, "The Response-to-Retention Hypothesis of Early Atherogenesis," *Arteriosclerosis, Thrombosis, and Vascular Biology* 15 (1995): 551–61.

11. Maria Gustafsson, Jan Borén, "Mechanism of Lipoprotein Retention by the Extracellular Matrix," *Current Opinion in Lipidology* 15, no. 5 (2004): 505–14.

12. Heart Protection Study Collaborative Group, "MRC/BHF Heart Protection Study of Antioxidant Vitamin Supplementation in 20,536 High-Risk Individuals: A Randomised Placebo-Controlled Trial," *Lancet* 360, no. 9326 (2002): 23–33.

13. Damon A. Bell, Amanda J. Hooper, John R. Burnett, "Mipomersen, an Antisense Apolipoprotein B Synthesis Inhibitor," *Expert Opinion in Investigational Drugs* 20, no. 2 (2011): 265–72.

14. Kuang-Yuh Chyu, Jan Nilsson, Prediman K. Shah, "Immune Mechanisms in Atherosclerosis and Potential for an Atherosclerosis Vaccine," *Discovery Medicine* 11, no. 60 (2011): 403–12.

15. J. P. Strong, H. C. McGill Jr., "The Pediatric Aspects of Atherosclerosis," *Journal of Atherosclerosis Research* 9, no. 3 (1969): 254–65.

16. Philip J. Barter et al., "Antiinflammatory Properties of HDL," *Circulation Research* 95, no. 8 (2004): 764–72.

17. David J. Gordon et al., "High-Density Lipoprotein Cholesterol and Cardiovascular Disease. Four Prospective American Studies," *Circulation* 79, no. 1 (1989): 8–15.

18. Valetin Fuster et al., "Atherothrombosis and High-Risk Plaque: Part I: Evolving Concepts," *Journal of the American College of Cardiology* 46, no. 6 (2005): 937–54.

19. Expert Panel on Detection, Evaluation, and Treatment of High Blood Cholesterol in Adults, "Executive Summary of the Third Report of the National Cholesterol Education Program (NCEP) Expert Panel on Detection, Evaluation, and Treatment of High Blood Cholesterol in Adults (Adult Treatment Panel III)," *Journal of the American Medical Association* 285, no. 19 (2001): 2486–97.

20. Cholesterol Treatment Trialists' (CTT) Collaboration, "Efficacy and Safety of More Intensive Lowering of LDL Cholesterol: A Meta-Analysis of Data from 170,000 Participants in 26 Randomised Trials," *Lancet* 376, no. 9753 (2010): 1670–81.

21. Jennifer G. Robinson et al., "Pleiotropic Effects of Statins: Benefit beyond Cholesterol Reduction? A Meta-Regression Analysis, *Journal of the American College of Cardiology* 46 (2005): 1855–62.

22. John R. Downs et al., "Primary Prevention of Acute Coronary Events with Lovastatin

in Men and Women with Average Cholesterol Levels: Results of AFCAPS/TexCAPS. Air Force/ Texas Coronary Atherosclerosis Prevention Study," *Journal of the American Medical Association* 279, no. 20 (1998): 1615–22.

23. Judith Hsia et al., "Cardiovascular Event Reduction and Adverse Events among Subjects Attaining Low-Density Lipoprotein Cholesterol < 50 mg/dL with Rosuvastatin," *Journal of the American College of Cardiology* 57, no. 16 (2011): 1666–75.

24. James H. O'Keefe Jr. et al., "Optimal Low-Density Lipoprotein Is 50 to 70 mg/dl: Lower Is Better and Physiologically Normal," *Journal of the American College of Cardiology* 43, no. 11 (2004): 2142–46.

25. Heart Protection Study Collaborative Group, "MRC/BHF Heart Protection Study of Cholesterol Lowering with Simvastatin in 20,536 High-Risk Individuals: A Randomized Placebo-Controlled Trial," *Lancet* 360 (2002): 7–22.

26. John C. LaRosa et al., "Intensive Lipid Lowering with Atorvastatin in Patients with Stable Coronary Disease," *New England Journal of Medicine* 352, no. 14 (2005): 1425–35.

27. Cholesterol Treatment Trialists' (CTT) Collaboration, "Efficacy and Safety," pp. 1670–81.

28. Paul M. Ridker et al., "Rosuvastatin to Prevent Vascular Events in Men and Women with Elevated C-Reactive Protein," *New England Journal of Medicine* 359, no. 21 (2008): 2195–207.

29. Paul M. Ridker et al., "Reduction in C-Reactive Protein and LDL Cholesterol and Cardiovascular Event Rates after Initiation of Rosuvastatin: A Prospective Study of the JUPITER Trial," *Lancet* 373, no. 9670 (2009): 1175–82.

30. Stuart P. Weisberg et al., "Obesity Is Associated with Macrophage Accumulation in Adipose Tissue," *Journal of Clinical Investigation* 112, no. 12 (2003): 1796–808.

31. Paul M. Ridker et al., "A Randomized Trial of Low-Dose Aspirin in the Primary Prevention of Cardiovascular Disease in Women," *New England Journal of Medicine* 352, no. 13 (2005): 1293–304.

32. Gavin J. Blake, Paul M. Ridker, "C-Reactive Protein and Other Inflammatory Risk Markers in Acute Coronary Syndromes," *Journal of the American College of Cardiology* 19, no. 4, supplement S (2003): 37S–42S.

33. Steven E. Nissen et al., "Effect of Very High-Intensity Statin Therapy on Regression of Coronary Atherosclerosis: The ASTEROID Trial," *Journal of the American Medical Association* 295, no. 13 (2006): 1556–65.

34. Stephen J. Nicholls et al., "Statins, High-Density Lipoprotein Cholesterol, and Regression of Coronary Atherosclerosis," *Journal of the American Medical Association* 297, no. 5 (2007): 499–508.

CHAPTER 2. RISK FACTORS AND PREVENTION IN THE 21st CENTURY

1. Salim Yusuf et al., "Effect of Potentially Modifiable Risk Factors Associated with Myocardial Infarction in 52 Countries (the INTERHEART Study): Case-Control Study," *Lancet* 364, no. 9438 (2004): 937–52.

2. Véronique L. Roger et al., "Heart Disease and Stroke Statistics 2011 Update: A Report from the American Heart Association," *Circulation* 123, no. 4 (2011): e18–209.

3. Earl S. Ford et al., "Explaining the Decrease in U.S. Deaths from Coronary Disease, 1980–2000," *New England Journal of Medicine* 356, no. 23 (2007): 2388–98.

4. Expert Panel on Detection, Evaluation, and Treatment of High Blood Cholesterol in Adults, "Executive Summary of the Third Report of the National Cholesterol Education Program (NCEP) Expert Panel on Detection, Evaluation, and Treatment of High Blood Cholesterol in Adults (Adult Treatment Panel III)," *Journal of the American Medical Association* 285, no. 19 (2001): 2486–97.

5. Paul M. Ridker et al., "Rosuvastatin for Primary Prevention among Individuals with Elevated High-Sensitivity C-Reactive Protein and 5% to 10% and 10% to 20% 10-Year Risk. Implications of the Justification for Use of Statins in Prevention: An Intervention Trial Evaluating Rosuvastatin (JUPITER) Trial for 'Intermediate Risk,'" *Circulation: Cardiovascular Quality and Outcomes* 3, no. 5 (2010): 447–52.

6. Roger et al., "Heart Disease and Stroke Statistics," pp. e18–209.

7. Scandinavian Simvastatin Survival Study Group, "Randomized Trial of Cholesterol Lowering in 4444 Patients with Coronary Artery Disease: The Scandinavian Simvastatin Survival Study (4S)," *Lancet* 344, no. 8934 (1994): 1383–89.

8. Frank M. Sacks et al., "The Effect of Pravastatin on Coronary Events after Myocardial Infarction in Patients with Average Cholesterol Levels: Cholesterol and Recurrent Events Trial Investigators," *New England Journal of Medicine* 335, no. 14 (1996): 1001–1009.

9. Jonathan C. Cohen et al., "Sequence Variations in PCSK9, Low LDL, and Protection against Coronary Heart Disease," *New England Journal of Medicine* 354, no. 12 (2006): 1264–72.

10. National Institutes of Health, National Heart, Lung, and Blood Institute, *Incidence and Prevalence: 2006 Chart Book on Cardiovascular and Lung Diseases* (Bethesda, MD: National Heart, Lung, and Blood Institute, 2006), http://www.nhlbi.nih.gov/resources/docs/06a_ip_chtbk.pdf (accessed September 23, 2011).

11. Jonathan Afilalo et al., "Statins for Secondary Prevention in Elderly Patients: A Hierarchical Bayesian Meta-Analysis," *Journal of the American College of Cardiology* 51, no. 1 (2008): 37–45.

12. Jacques E. Rossouw et al., "Risks and Benefits of Estrogen Plus Progestin in Healthy Postmenopausal Women: Principal Results from the Women's Health Initiative Randomized Controlled Trial," *Journal of the American Medical Association* 288, no. 3 (2002): 321–33.

13. William F. Enos, Robert H. Holmes, James Beyer, "Coronary Disease among United States Soldiers Killed in Action in Korea: Preliminary Report," *Journal of the American Medical Association* 152, no. 12 (1953): 1090–93.

14. Antonio M. Gotto Jr., Henry J. Pownall, *Manual of Lipid Disorders: Reducing the Risk for Coronary Heart Disease*, 3rd ed. (Philadelphia: Lippincott Williams & Wilkins, 2003).

15. Expert Panel on Detection, Evaluation, and Treatment of High Blood Cholesterol in Adults, "Executive Summary," pp. 2486–97.

16. National Center for Health Statistics, *Health, United States, 2010: With Special Feature on Death and Dying* (Hyattsville, MD: US Department of Health and Human Services, 2011), p. 25, http://www.cdc.gov/nchs/data/hus/hus10.pdf (accessed September 23, 2011).

17. Roger et al., "Heart Disease and Stroke Statistics," pp. e18–209.

18. Scott M. Grundy et al., "Implications of Recent Clinical Trials for the National Cholesterol Education Program Adult Treatment Panel III Guidelines," *Circulation* 110, no. 2 (2004): 227–39.

19. Gavin J. Blake et al., "Low-Density Lipoprotein Particle Concentration and Size as Determined by Nuclear Magnetic Resonance Spectroscopy as Predictors of Cardiovascular Disease in Women," *Circulation* 106, no. 15 (2002): 1930–37.

20. Antonio M. Gotto Jr. *Contemporary Diagnosis and Management of Lipid Disorders*, 4th ed. (Newtown, PA: Handbooks in Health Care, 2008) pp. 184–255.

21. Cholesterol Treatment Trialists' (CTT) Collaboration, "Efficacy and Safety of More Intensive Lowering of LDL Cholesterol: A Meta-Analysis of Data from 170,000 Participants in 26 Randomised Trials," *Lancet* 376, no. 9753 (2010): 1670–81.

22. Jane Armitage, "The Safety of Statins in Clinical Practice," *Lancet* 370, no. 9601 (2007): 1781–90.

23. US Food and Drug Administration, "FDA Drug Safety Communication: New Restrictions, Contraindications, and Dose Limitations for Zocor (Simvastatin) to Reduce the Risk of Muscle Injury," http://www.fda.gov/Drugs/DrugSafety/ucm256581.htm (accessed September 21, 2011).

24. Naveed Sattar et al., "Statins and Risk of Incident Diabetes: A Collaborative Meta-Analysis of Randomised Statin Trials," *Lancet* 375, no. 9716 (2010): 735–42.

25. John J. Kastelein et al., "Simvastatin with or without Ezetimibe in Familial Hypercholesterolemia," *New England Journal of Medicine* 358, no. 14 (2008): 1431–43; Anne B. Rossebø et al., "Intensive Lipid Lowering with Simvastatin and Ezetimibe in Aortic Stenosis," *New England Journal of Medicine* 359, no. 13 (2008): 1343–56; Todd C. Villines et al., "The ARBITER 6-HALTS Trial (Arterial Biology for the Investigation of the Treatment Effects of Reducing Cholesterol 6-HDL and LDL Treatment Strategies in Atherosclerosis): Final Results and the Impact of Medication Adherence, Dose, and Treatment Duration," *Journal of the American College of Cardiology* 55, no. 24 (2010): 2721–26.

26. Colin Baigent et al., "The Effects of Lowering LDL Cholesterol with Simvastatin Plus

Ezetimibe in Patients with Chronic Kidney Disease (Study of Heart and Renal Protection): A Randomized Placebo-Controlled Trial," *Lancet* 377, no. 9784 (2011): 2181–92.

27. Roger et al., "Heart Disease and Stroke Statistics," pp. e18–209.

28. Aram V. Chobanian et al., "The Seventh Report of the Joint National Committee on Prevention, Detection, Evaluation, and Treatment of High Blood Pressure: The JNC 7 Report," *Journal of the American Medical Association* 289, no. 19 (2003): 2560–72.

29. National Center for Health Statistics, *Health*, p. 25.

30. Roger et al., "Heart Disease and Stroke Statistics," pp. e18–209.

31. J. Peralez Gunn et al., "Sodium Intake among Adults—United States, 2005–2006," *Morbidity and Mortality Weekly Report* 59, no. 24 (June 25, 2010): 746–49.

32. National High Blood Pressure Education Program, *The Seventh Report of the Joint National Committee on Prevention, Detection, Evaluation, and Treatment of High Blood Pressure* (Bethesda, MD: National Heart, Lung, and Blood Institute, 2004).

33. Lionel H. Opie, Bernard J. Gersh, *Drugs for the Heart*, 7th ed. (Philadelphia: Saunders, 2009), pp. 88–111.

34. Peter Sever et al., "Potential Synergy between Lipid-Lowering and Blood-Pressure-Lowering in the Anglo-Scandinavian Cardiac Outcomes Trial," *European Heart Journal* 27, no. 24 (2006): 2982–88.

35. Centers for Disease Control, "Tobacco Use: Targeting the Nation's Leading Killer at a Glance 2011," http://www.cdc.gov/chronicdisease/resources/publications/aag/osh.htm (accessed September 23, 2011).

36. American Heart Association, "Smoking: Do You Really Know the Risks?" http://www.heart.org/HEARTORG/GettingHealthy/QuitSmoking/QuittingSmoking/Smoking-Do-you-really-know-the-risks_UCM_322718_Article.jsp (accessed September 23, 2011).

37. US Food and Drug Administration, "Public Health Advisory: FDA Requires New Boxed Warning for the Smoking Cessation Drugs Chantix and Zyban," http://www.fda.gov/Drugs/DrugSafety/PostmarketDrugSafetyInformationforPatientsandProviders/DrugSafetyInformation forHeathcareProfessionals/PublicHealthAdvisories/ucm169988.htm (accessed September 23, 2011).

38. American Cancer Society, "Stay Away from Tobacco," http://www.cancer.org/Healthy/StayAwayfromTobacco/index (accessed September 23, 2011).

39. Centers for Disease Control and Prevention, *National Diabetes Fact Sheet: National Estimates and General Information on Diabetes and Prediabetes in the United States, 2011* (Atlanta: US Department of Health and Human Services, Centers for Disease Control and Prevention, 2011), http://www.cdc.gov/diabetes/pubs/pdf/ndfs_2011.pdf (accessed September 23, 2011).

40. Charles M. Alexander et al., "NCEP-Defined Metabolic Syndrome, Diabetes, and Prevalence of Coronary Heart Disease among NHANES III Participants Age 50 Years and Older," *Diabetes* 52, no. 5 (2003): 1210–14.

41. Antonio M. Gotto Jr., "Cardiologist's Role in Improving Glucose Control and Global

Cardiovascular Risk in Patients with Type 2 Diabetes Mellitus," *American Journal of Cardiology* 99, no. 4 (2007): 3–5.

42. Earl S. Ford, Guixiang Zhao, Chaoyang Li, "Pre-Diabetes and the Risk for Cardiovascular Disease: A Systematic Review of the Evidence," *Journal of the American College of Cardiology* 55, no. 13 (2010): 1310–17.

43. ACCORD Study Group, "Effects of Intensive Glucose Lowering in Type 2 Diabetes," *New England Journal of Medicine* 358, no. 924 (2008): 2545–59.

44. ADVANCE Collaborative Group, "Intensive Blood Glucose Control and Vascular Outcomes in Patients with Type 2 Diabetes," *New England Journal of Medicine* 358, no. 24 (2008): 2560–72; William Duckworth et al., "Glucose Control and Vascular Complications in Veterans with Type 2 Diabetes," *New England Journal of Medicine* 360, no. 2 (2009): 129–39.

45. Cholesterol Treatment Trialists' (CTT) Collaborators, "Efficacy of Cholesterol-Lowering Therapy in 18,686 People with Diabetes in 14 Randomised Trials of Statins: A Meta-Analysis," *Lancet* 371 (2008): 117–25.

46. Francesco Rubino, "Is Type 2 Diabetes an Operable Intestinal Disease?" *Diabetes Care* 31, Supplement 2 (2008): S290–96.

47. Alice H. Lichtenstein et al., "Diet and Lifestyle Recommendations Revision 2006: A Scientific Statement from the American Heart Association Nutrition Committee," *Circulation* 114 (2006): 82–96.

48. Ibid.

49. Youfa Wang, May A. Beydoun, "The Obesity Epidemic in the United States—Gender, Age, Socioeconomic, Racial/Ethnic, and Geographic Characteristics: A Systematic Review and Meta-Regression Analysis," *Epidemiologic Reviews* 29, no. 1 (2007): 6–28.

50. Roger et al., "Heart Disease and Stroke Statistics," pp. e18–209.

51. Ibid.

52. Expert Panel on Detection, Evaluation, and Treatment of High Blood Cholesterol in Adults, "Executive Summary," pp. 2486–97.

53. US Food and Drug Administration, "Meridia (Sibutramine): Market Withdrawal Due to Risk of Serious Cardiovascular Events," http://www.fda.gov/safety/medwatch/safetyinformation/safetyalertsforhumanmedicalproducts/ucm228830.htm (accessed September 23, 2011).

54. Robert Allan, Jeffrey Fisher, *Heart and Mind: The Practice of Cardiac Psychology*, 2nd ed. (Washington, DC: American Psychological Association, 2011).

55. Clifton Fadiman and André Bernard, eds., *Bartlett's Book of Anecdotes* (Boston: Little, Brown, 2000), p. 282.

56. Murray A. Mittelman et al., "Triggering of Acute Myocardial Infarction Onset by Episodes of Anger: Determinants of Myocardial Infarction Onset Study Investigators," *Circulation* 92, no. 7 (1995): 1720–25.

57. Jonathan Leor, W. Kenneth Poole, Robert A. Kloner, "Sudden Cardiac Death Triggered by an Earthquake," *New England Journal of Medicine* 334, no. 7 (1996): 413–19.

58. Daniel Weisenberg, Simcha R. Meisel, Daniel David, "Sudden Death among the Israeli Civilian Population During the Gulf War—Incidence and Mechanisms," *Israel Journal of Medical Sciences*, 32, no. 2 (1996): 95–99.

59. Dominique Lecomte, Paul Fornes, Guy Nicolas, "Stressful Events as a Trigger of Sudden Death: A Study of 43 Medico-Legal Autopsy Cases," *Forensic Science International* 79, no. 1 (1996): 1–10.

60. Mats Gulliksson et al., "Randomized Controlled Trial of Cognitive Behavioral Therapy vs. Standard Treatment to Prevent Recurrent Cardiovascular Events in Patients with Coronary Heart Disease: Secondary Prevention in Uppsala Primary Health Care Project (SUPRIM)," *Archives of Internal Medicine* 171, no. 2 (2011): 134–40.

61. Roger et al., "Heart Disease and Stroke Statistics," pp. e18–209.

62. Ibid.

63. Andrew G. Bostom et al., "Nonfasting Plasma Total Homocysteine Levels and All-Cause and Cardiovascular Disease Mortality in Elderly Framingham Men and Women," *Archives of Internal Medicine* 159, no. 10 (1999): 1077–80; Andrew G. Bostom et al., "Nonfasting Plasma Total Homocysteine Levels and Stroke Incidence in Elderly Persons: The Framingham Study," *Annals of Internal Medicine* 131, no. 5 (1999): 352–55; Meir J. Stampfer et al., "A Prospective Study of Plasma Homocyst(e)ine and Risk of Myocardial Infarction in US Physicians," *Journal of the American Medical Association* 268, no. 7 (1992): 877–81.

64. James F. Toole et al., "Lowering Homocysteine in Patients with Ischemic Stroke to Prevent Recurrent Stroke, Myocardial Infarction, and Death: The Vitamin Intervention for Stroke Prevention (VISP) Randomized Controlled Trial," *Journal of the American Medical Association* 291, no. 5 (2004): 565–75; Eva Lonn et al., "Homocysteine Lowering with Folic Acid and B Vitamins in Vascular Disease," *New England Journal of Medicine* 354 (2006): 1567–77; Kaare H. Bonaa et al., "Homocysteine Lowering and Cardiovascular Events after Acute Myocardial Infarction," *New England Journal of Medicine* 354 (2006): 1578–88.

65. David J. Becker et al., "Red Yeast Rice for Dyslipidemia in Statin-Intolerant Patients: A Randomized Trial," *Annals of Internal Medicine* 150, no. 12 (2009): 830–39.

CHAPTER 3. DETERMINING YOUR CARDIAC HEALTH

1. Vijay Nambi et al., "Carotid Intima-Media Thickness and Presence or Absence of Plaque Improves Prediction of Coronary Heart Disease Risk: The ARIC (Atherosclerosis Risk in Communities) Study," *Journal of the American College of Cardiology* 55, no. 15 (2010): 1600–1607.

2. George M. Schuetz et al., "Meta-Analysis: Noninvasive Coronary Angiography Using Computed Tomography versus Magnetic Resonance Imaging," *Annals of Internal Medicine* 152, no. 3 (2010): 167–77.

3. American College of Radiology and Radiological Society of North America, "Patient Safety: Radiation Exposure in X-Ray and CT Examinations," http://www.radiologyinfo.org/en/safety/index.cfm?pg=sfty_xray (accessed September 26, 2011).

4. Andrew J. Einstein et al., "Radiation Dose to Patients from Cardiac Diagnostic Imaging," *Circulation* 116 (2007): 1290–305.

5. Nikolaos Alexopoulos, Paolo Raggi, "Calcification in Atherosclerosis," *Nature Reviews Cardiology* 6, no. 11 (2009): 681–88.

6. American College of Radiology, "Patient Safety."

7. Ibid.

8. Einstein et al., "Radiation Dose," pp. 1290–305.

CHAPTER 4. ATHEROSCLEROTIC VASCULAR DISEASE

1. Véronique L. Roger et al., "Heart Disease and Stroke Statistics 2011 Update: A Report from the American Heart Association," *Circulation* 123, no. 4 (2011): e18–209.

2. Robert O. Bonow et al., eds., *Braunwald's Heart Disease: A Textbook of Cardiovascular Medicine*, 9th ed. (Philadelphia: Saunders, 2011), pp. 1049–1391; James T. Willerson et al., eds., *Cardiovascular Medicine*, 3rd ed. (London: Springer-Verlag, 2007), pp. 911–78, 995–1134.

3. Roger et al., "Heart Disease and Stroke Statistics," pp. e18–209.

4. Christopher P. Cannon et al., "Intensive versus Moderate Lipid Lowering with Statins after Acute Coronary Syndromes," *New England Journal of Medicine* 350, no. 15 (2004): 1495–1504.

5. Roger et al., "Heart Disease and Stroke Statistics," pp. e18–209.

CHAPTER 5. TREATING ATHEROSCLEROTIC DISEASE IN THE 21st CENTURY

1. Robert O. Bonow et al. eds., *Braunwald's Heart Disease: A Textbook of Cardiovascular Medicine*, 9th ed. (Philadelphia: Saunders, 2011), pp. 1049–1391; James T. Willerson et al., eds., *Cardiovascular Medicine*, 3rd ed. (London: Springer-Verlag, 2007), pp. 911–78, 995–1134; Lionel H. Opie, Bernard J. Gersh, *Drugs for the Heart*, 7th ed. (Philadelphia: Saunders, 2009), pp. 1–87, 112–59, 293–34, 388–458.

2. Gilles R. Dagenais et al., "Angiotensin-Converting-Enzyme Inhibitors in Stable Vascular Disease without Left Ventricular Systolic Dysfunction or Heart Failure: A Combined Analysis of Three Trials," *Lancet* 368, no. 9535 (2006): 581–88.

3. Antithrombotic Trialists' Collaboration, "Aspirin in the Primary and Secondary Prevention of Vascular Disease: Collaborative Meta-Analysis of Individual Participant Data from Randomised Trials," *Lancet* 373, no. 9678 (2009): 1849–60.

4. William E. Boden et al., "Optimal Medical Therapy with or without PCI for Stable Coronary Disease," *New England Journal of Medicine* 356, no. 15 (2007): 1506–16.

CHAPTER 6. ARRHYTHMIAS

1. Robert O. Bonow et al., eds., *Braunwald's Heart Disease: A Textbook of Cardiovascular Medicine*, 9th ed. (Philadelphia: Saunders, 2011), pp. 653–896; James T. Willerson et al., eds., *Cardiovascular Medicine*, 3rd ed. (London: Springer-Verlag, 2007), pp. 1925–2176; Lionel H. Opie, Bernard J. Gersh, *Drugs for the Heart*, 7th ed. (Philadelphia: Saunders, 2009), pp. 235–92, 388–408.

2. Simon de Denus et al., "Rate vs. Rhythm Control in Patients with Atrial Fibrillation: A Meta-Analysis," *Archives of Internal Medicine* 165, no. 3 (2005): 258–62.

CHAPTER 7. HEART FAILURE

1. Robert O. Bonow et al., eds., *Braunwald's Heart Disease: A Textbook of Cardiovascular Medicine*, 9th ed. (Philadelphia: Saunders, 2011), pp. 458–643; James T. Willerson et al., eds., *Cardiovascular Medicine*, 3rd ed. (London: Springer-Verlag, 2007), pp. 1379–478; Lionel H. Opie, Bernard J. Gersh, *Drugs for the Heart*, 7th ed. (Philadelphia: Saunders, 2009), pp. 160–97, 388–408.

2. Véronique L. Roger et al., "Heart Disease and Stroke Statistics 2011 Update: A Report from the American Heart Association," *Circulation* 123, no. 4 (2011): e18–209.

3. Carol J. DeFrances et al., "2006 National Hospital Discharge Survey," *National Health Statistics Reports* 5 (2008): 1–20.

4. Roger et al., "Heart Disease and Stroke Statistics," pp. e18–209.

5. Anne L. Taylor et al., "Combination of Isosorbide Dinitrate and Hydralazine in Blacks with Heart Failure," *New England Journal of Medicine* 351, no. 20 (2004): 2049–57.

6. Eric A. Rose et al., "Long-Term Use of a Left Ventricular Assist Device for End-Stage Heart Failure," *New England Journal of Medicine* 345, no. 20 (2001): 1435–43.

7. Finlay A. McAlister et al., "Cardiac Resynchronization Therapy and Implantable Cardiac Defibrillators in Left Ventricular Systolic Dysfunction," *Evidence Report/Technology Assessment* No. 152 (Prepared by the University of Alberta Evidence-Based Practice Center under Contract No. 290-02-0023), AHRQ Publication No. 07-E009 (Rockville, MD: Agency for Healthcare Research and Quality, 2007).

8. Kosmas I. Paraskevas, "Application of Statins in Cardiothoracic Surgery: More Than Just Lipid-Lowering," *European Journal of Cardiothoracic Surgery* 33, no. 3 (2008): 377–90.

CHAPTER 8. VALVULAR HEART DISEASE

1. Robert O. Bonow et al., eds., *Braunwald's Heart Disease: A Textbook of Cardiovascular Medicine*, 9th ed. (Philadelphia: Saunders, 2011), pp. 1468–594, 1628–37; James T. Willerson et al., eds., *Cardiovascular Medicine*, 3rd ed. (London: Springer-Verlag, 2007), pp. 369–430, 557–92.

2. Anne B. Rossebø et al., "Intensive Lipid Lowering with Simvastatin and Ezetimibe in Aortic Stenosis," *New England Journal of Medicine* 359, no. 13 (2008): 1343–56; Alessandro Parolari et al., "Do Statins Improve Outcomes and Delay the Progression of Non-Rheumatic Calcific Aortic Stenosis?" *Heart* 97, no. 7 (2011): 523–29.

3. Walter Wilson et al., "Prevention of Infective Endocarditis: Guidelines from the American Heart Association," *Circulation* 116 (2007): 1736–54.

4. Martin B. Leon et al., "Transcatheter Aortic-Valve Implantation for Aortic Stenosis in Patients Who Cannot Undergo Surgery," *New England Journal of Medicine* 363, no. 17 (2010): 1597–607.

5. Ted Feldman et al., "Percutaneous Repair or Surgery for Mitral Regurgitation," *New England Journal of Medicine* 364, no. 15 (2011): 1395–406.

CHAPTER 9. THE FUTURE OF CARDIOVASCULAR MEDICINE

1. Ali J. Marian, "The Personal Genome and the Practice of Cardiovascular Medicine," *Methodist DeBakey Cardiovascular Journal* 6, no. 4 (Nov 2010–Jan 2011): 13–20.

2. Heribert Schunkert et al., "Large-Scale Association Analysis Identifies 13 New Susceptibility Loci for Coronary Artery Disease," *Nature Genetics* 43, no. 4 (2011): 333–38.

3. Jonathan C. Cohen et al., "Sequence Variations in PCSK9, Low LDL, and Protection against Coronary Heart Disease," *New England Journal of Medicine* 354, no. 12 (2006): 1264–72.

4. Ruth McPherson et al., "A Common Allele on Chromosome 9 Associated with Coronary Heart Disease," *Science* 316, no. 5831 (2007): 1488–91; Heribert Schunkert et al., "Repeated Replication and a Prospective Meta-Analysis of the Association between Chromosome 9p21.3 and Coronary Artery Disease," *Circulation* 117, no. 13 (2008): 1675–84.

5. US Food and Drug Administration, "FDA Approves Updated Warfarin (Coumadin) Prescribing Information: New Genetic Information May Help Providers Improve Initial Dosing

Estimates of the Anticoagulant for Individual Patients," http://www.fda.gov/NewsEvents/Newsroom/PressAnnouncements/2007/ucm108967.htm (accessed September 26, 2011).

6. Robert S. Epstein et al., "Warfarin Genotyping Reduces Hospitalization Rates Results from the MM-WES (Medco-Mayo Warfarin Effectiveness Study)," *Journal of the American College of Cardiology* 55, no. 25 (2010): 2804–12.

7. US Food and Drug Administration, "FDA Drug Safety Communication: Reduced Effectiveness of Plavix (Clopidogrel) in Patients Who Are Poor Metabolizers of the Drug," http://www.fda.gov/drugs/drugsafety/PostmarketDrugSafetyInformationforPatientsandProviders/ucm203888.htm (accessed September 26, 2011).

8. SEARCH Collaborative Group, "SLCO1B1 Variants and Statin-Induced Myopathy—A Genomewide Study," *New England Journal of Medicine* 359 (2008): 789–99; John F. Thompson et al., "An Association Study of 43 SNPs in 16 Candidate Genes with Atorvastatin Response," *Pharmacogenomics Journal* 5, no. 6 (2005): 352–58.

9. Sharon Cresci et al., "Clinical and Genetic Modifiers of Long-Term Survival in Heart Failure," *Journal of the American College of Cardiology* 54, no. 5 (2009): 432–44.

10. Marja Hedman, Juha Hartikainen, and Seppo Yla-Herttuala, "Progress and Prospects: Hurdles to Cardiovascular Gene Therapy Clinical Trials," *Gene Therapy* 18, no. 8 (2011): 743–49.

11. Kazutoshi Takahashi and Shinya Yamanaka, "Induction of Pluripotent Stem Cells from Mouse Embryonic and Adult Fibroblast Cultures by Defined Factors," *Cell* 126, no. 4 (2006): 663–76; Junying Yu et al., "Induced Pluripotent Stem Cell Lines Derived from Human Somatic Cells," *Science* 318, no. 5858 (2007): 1917–20; Kazutoshi Takahashi et al., "Induction of Pluripotent Stem Cells from Adult Human Fibroblasts by Defined Factors," *Cell* 131, no. 5 (2007): 861–72.

12. Vincent F. M. Segers and Richard T. Lee, "Stem-Cell Therapy for Cardiac Disease," *Nature* 451, no. 7181 (2008): 937–42.

ADDITIONAL RESOURCES

F or more information on heart disease, its prevention, and its treatment, below is a list of useful websites and organizations.

American Heart Association
http://www.heart.org

American Stroke Association
http://www.strokeassociation.org

Centers for Disease Control and Prevention
http://www.cdc.gov/heartdisease/

National Heart, Lung, and Blood Institute
http://www.nhlbi.nih.gov

National Institute of Neurological Disorders and Stroke
http://www.ninds.nih.gov

National Library of Medicine's Medline Plus
http://www.nlm.nih.gov/medlineplus/

GLOSSARY

ACE inhibitors. A short name for angiotensin-converting enzyme inhibitors, which are medications that improve blood flow by dilating blood vessels. They are used to treat high blood pressure; to treat and prevent heart failure, particularly of the left ventricle; and to protect against future cardiovascular events in patients with coronary heart disease.

acute coronary syndrome (ACS). Refers to unstable angina or a heart attack.

adventitia. The outermost layer of the arterial wall.

aneurysm. A balloon-like sac formed by the stretching of the walls of an artery.

angina. Chest pain resulting from decreased blood flow to the heart, most often due to atherosclerotic disease of the coronary arteries.

angina, stable. Angina that occurs only during exercise or stress, typically lasts about five minutes or less, and usually disappears after rest or taking nitroglycerin.

angina, unstable. Angina that occurs at rest or with progressively less intense levels of exertion, typically lasts longer than twenty minutes, and is often not relieved with rest or nitroglycerin.

angina, variant. Also called **Prinzmetal's angina.** An uncommon form of angina caused by a localized spasm of a coronary artery.

angiography. Visualization of the inside of arteries, veins, or the chambers of the heart. It is traditionally performed with cardiac catheterization and x-rays, and newer techniques incorporate CT and MRI imaging.

angiotensin II. A hormone that causes blood vessels to constrict.

angiotensin receptor blocker (ARB). Drugs that act on the receptor for angiotensin II to widen blood vessels. Often prescribed to individuals intolerant of ACE inhibitors.

ankle/brachial index (ABI). The ratio of the systolic blood pressure at the ankle to the systolic blood pressure in the arm. The ratio, which should normally be 1.0 or greater, can help detect peripheral artery disease in the legs.

anticoagulant drugs. Also called **antithrombotics**. Drugs, including heparin, thrombin inhibitors, and warfarin, that prevent blood from clotting by interfering with the production or activity of a protein called thrombin.

anti-ischemic drugs. Drugs, including nitrates, beta-blockers, and calcium channel blockers, used to treat symptoms of coronary heart disease. They reduce the demand for oxygen by the heart and increase blood flow to the heart, often decreasing the chest pain of angina.

antiplatelet drugs. Drugs, including aspirin, ADP receptor antagonists, cilostazol, and glycoprotein IIb/IIIa inhibitors, that prevent the activation of platelets in the blood, thereby preventing blood clot formation.

aorta. The main artery carrying blood from the heart to the rest of the body.

aortic regurgitation. A valvular disease in which the aortic valve does not close tightly, allowing blood to flow backward from the aorta to the left ventricle of the heart.

aortic stenosis. Narrowing of the aortic valve opening that connects the left ventricle and the aorta.

aortic valve. The valve separating the left ventricle of the heart from the aorta.

apolipoprotein B. Also called **apo B**. A major protein component of LDL, IDL, and VLDL that is associated with increased risk for coronary heart disease.

arrhythmia. Any variation from the normal rhythm of the heartbeat.

artery. A vessel that carries blood from the heart to the tissues of the body, ending in small branches called arterioles, which, in turn, branch to form the capillaries.

atherogenic dyslipidemia. Also called the **lipid triad**. A lipid profile associated with increased atherosclerosis and commonly found in people with diabetes and the metabolic syndrome. Characterized by high triglycerides, low HDL-C, and small dense LDL particles.

atherosclerosis. Also called **atherosclerotic vascular disease**. A disease of the arteries in which lipids are deposited within the arterial wall and form plaques. It is associated with inflammation, growth of smooth muscle cells, and other changes in the arterial wall, leading to a hardening and narrowing of the arteries. It is the most common cause of heart attacks and strokes.

atherosclerotic plaque. Also called **atherosclerotic lesions.** Deposits of lipids (fatty material) and other substances within the arterial wall, often encased by a thin layer of fibrous cells, which may progress to narrow or block an artery. Plaques may also rupture to form a blood clot.

atria. Singular, **atrium.** Upper chambers of the heart that receive blood from the lungs and body.

atrial fibrillation. A type of arrhythmia in which the atria quiver without beating effectively, with fast and irregular contractions of the ventricles.

atrial flutter. A type of arrhythmia in which the atria beat very quickly. The ventricles may also beat quickly and in a coordinated pattern.

atrioventricular (AV) node. The heart's secondary pacemaker. It receives impulses from the sinoatrial node and transmits them to another part of the heart's electrical conduction system called the bundle branches, which triggers the contraction of the ventricles.

beta-blockers. Another name for **beta-adrenergic antagonists,** a class of drugs that slow the heart rate and decrease the force of the heart's pumping action. It has many uses, including treatment of high blood pressure, management of heart failure, treatment of arrhythmias, protection of the heart in patients following a heart attack, and reduction of chest pain in patients with angina and acute coronary syndromes.

bile acid resins. Also called **resins** and **bile acid sequestrants.** A class of drugs that lower LDL-C levels by increasing the amount of cholesterol that is excreted as bile acids from the intestines.

bradycardia. A slow resting heart rate, less than sixty beats per minute.

bruit. A swishing noise produced by blood as it rushes through an artery narrowed by an obstruction.

calcium channel blocker. A class of drugs that relax and widen blood vessels and that decrease the resistance from blood flow throughout the body's vessels. Used to treat high blood pressure, stable angina, variant angina, and arrhythmias. May be administered in patients during acute coronary syndromes or following a heart attack if they are unable to take beta-blockers.

cardiac allograft vasculopathy (CAV). Also called **graft coronary artery**

disease. A form of accelerated atherosclerosis that develops in a transplanted heart.

cardiac arrest. Cessation of heart function.

cardiac catheterization. Insertion of a catheter through an artery or vein, often in the groin area, which is then directed into the heart in order to visualize its arteries, chambers, or valves. May be performed for diagnostic purposes and as part of a percutaneous intervention.

cardiac event monitor. Similar to a Holter® monitor, a portable electrocardiography device that can be worn outside of the doctor's office for extended periods of time (weeks or months) in order to detect arrhythmias.

cardiac rehabilitation. A formal program consisting of education, counseling, risk factor modification, and progressive exercise, designed for patients recovering from a coronary event or cardiovascular surgery.

cardiac resynchronization therapy. Also known as **biventricular pacing**. A form of therapy for heart failure that uses a specialized pacemaker to recoordinate the contractions of both ventricles. The device may incorporate a defibrillator.

cardiomyopathy. A group of diseases often characterized by enlargement of the heart; some forms result in a thickened or stiffened heart muscle.

cardiopulmonary bypass. Also used to refer to the **heart-lung machine**. During open-heart surgery, the heart is stopped, and the circulation is maintained with the use of the heart-lung machine, which oxygenates the blood and removes carbon dioxide from it.

cardiovascular disease. A general class of diseases affecting the heart, arteries, and veins. It includes coronary heart disease, peripheral artery disease, stroke, arrhythmias, heart failure, and valvular disease, as well as many other conditions.

cardioversion. Restoration of a normal heartbeat by administration of an electric shock or a drug.

carotid endarterectomy. A surgical procedure in which the carotid artery in the neck is opened and the atherosclerotic plaque is peeled away from the arterial wall.

catheter. A long, extremely narrow tube used in cardiac diagnostic and therapeutic procedures to introduce fluids or devices into the blood vessels.

catheter ablation. A procedure to treat arrhythmias using a catheter to deactivate an area of heart tissue with radiofrequency energy. Sites responsible for arrhythmias are identified by a prior electrophysiology study.

cholesterol. A type of lipid or fat. The body gets cholesterol both by making it and from diet.

cholesterol absorption inhibitor. A class of drug that lowers LDL-C levels by decreasing the absorption of dietary cholesterol in the intestines. Ezetimibe is the only drug in this class and is often used in patients who are intolerant of statins, or in combination with statins in patients who require large LDL-C reductions.

cholesteryl ester. The primary form of cholesterol transported in the blood.

chylomicron. A large lipoprotein in the blood that is produced in the intestine from triglycerides and cholesterol obtained in the diet. Chylomicrons deliver free fatty acids and triglycerides to cells and are not associated with the development of atherosclerosis.

chylomicron remnant. Partially digested chylomicron. May accelerate atherosclerosis.

collateral circulation. The development of connections around an obstruction to blood flow by the growth of small arteries above and below the obstruction. This is nature's method of compensating for obstruction in blood flow.

computed tomography. Also called **CT** or **CAT scanning.** A noninvasive technique to examine the body's internal structures using x-rays in which three-dimensional images are created by computer reconstructions of two-dimensional views.

congestive heart failure. May be used synonymously with **heart failure.** A form of heart failure characterized by fluid retention in the lungs and edema of the legs.

contrast agent. A substance introduced into the body to enhance visualization during imaging tests.

coronary artery bypass grafting (CABG). Also called **bypass surgery.** A surgical procedure in which a graft, typically constructed from a patient's own blood vessel, is attached to an artery above and below the site of obstruction to provide normal blood flow to the diseased vessel.

coronary artery disease. Often used interchangeably with **coronary heart disease.** It is the most common form of heart disease and can lead to angina or a heart attack. It arises due to atherosclerotic plaque growth within the coronary arteries surrounding the heart.

coronary calcium scan. A noninvasive diagnostic test using ultrafast computed tomography to detect the presence of calcium deposits in the coronary arteries (can be a sign of atherosclerosis, but also associated with aging). The coronary calcium score is used by doctors to help predict a patient's risk of developing future heart disease.

C-reactive protein. A sign or marker of inflammation throughout the body associated with increased risk for coronary heart disease. May be used to identify people at increased risk for heart disease despite having low LDL-C levels.

creatine kinase. An enzyme that indicates muscle damage and is used to diagnose statin-related muscle disease (myopathy).

critical limb ischemia. A severe form of peripheral artery disease in which pain in the legs is felt at rest. Can lead to gangrene and loss of limb.

cyanosis. A clinical condition characterized by a bluish appearance caused by a lack of oxygen in the blood.

defibrillation. Termination of an extremely rapid, irregular, and potentially fatal heartbeat, usually by electric shock.

diastole. The phase of the heart's cycle during which it relaxes and its chambers fill with blood.

diastolic blood pressure. The lower number in a blood pressure reading, observed during diastole, when the heart fills with blood.

diastolic heart failure. Type of heart failure due to an impairment in the heart's ability to relax and fill sufficiently with blood.

direct renin inhibitor. A new class of antihypertensive medication that blocks the enzyme renin in the kidney, resulting in relaxation and widening of blood vessels.

diuretic. A drug that promotes excretion of urine. Often used to treat hypertension and manage symptoms of heart failure.

dyslipidemia. A lipid disorder, such as hypercholesterolemia and hypertriglyceridemia.

dyspnea. Labored or difficult breathing.

echocardiography. A method of imaging and recording the motion of the wall and internal structures of the heart using ultrasound. The standard method is **transthoracic echocardiography,** with sound waves directed through the chest; with **transesophageal echocardiography,** sound waves are emitted from a device placed inside the patient's esophagus.

edema. Fluid accumulation within the body's tissues.

ejection fraction. The part, or fraction, of the blood in the ventricles that is ejected with each heartbeat.

electrocardiography (ECG or EKG). Recording of the electrical impulses of the heart in a two-dimensional waveform.

electrolyte. A salt or mineral that helps regulate various bodily processes such as fluid balance. Includes sodium, potassium, magnesium, and calcium.

electrophysiology study. A diagnostic test of the heart's electrical conduction system in order to identify the source of an arrhythmia and to evaluate and determine the course of treatment.

embolism. The sudden blocking of a blood vessel by an embolus.

embolus. A blood clot or other matter that travels through the bloodstream to lodge in another vessel and obstruct the circulation.

endothelium. The innermost layer of cells lining a blood vessel.

exercise stress test. A type of diagnostic test in which patients may walk on a treadmill, pedal a stationary cycle, or receive drugs that stimulate the heart while physicians use electrocardiography, echocardiography, nuclear imaging, or MRI to study heart function and coronary artery blood supply.

fasting plasma glucose (FPG). A blood test used to diagnose diabetes that measures blood sugar levels after fasting for at least eight hours. People with **impaired fasting glucose** have prediabetes and are at increased risk for developing diabetes.

fatty acid. A type of simple lipid derived from animal and vegetable fats and oils. **Free fatty acids** are used by muscles for energy or can be converted to triglycerides and stored as fat. **Omega-3 fatty acids** are found primarily in fish and have beneficial cardiovascular effects. *Trans* **fatty acids** used in commercially prepared foods increase risk for coronary heart disease.

fatty streak. A small, flat, yellowish patch in the artery wall that appears to be the earliest lesion in the development of atherosclerosis. It can be found in young children.

fibrates. A class of drugs that raise HDL-C and lower triglyceride levels through various mechanisms. Also increase the size of small dense LDL.

fibrillation. Uncoordinated, irregular contractions of the heart that do not effectively pump blood and produce a "quivering" heart muscle.

fibrin. A protein that is formed by the action of thrombin to produce a blood clot.

fibrinogen. A protein found in the blood that plays a role in the blood-clotting process and is associated with increased risk for coronary heart disease.

foam cell. A component of fatty streaks, an early sign of atherosclerosis. These cells result when macrophages (specialized white blood cells) ingest LDL and become filled with lipid.

gene therapy. The process of introducing genetic material, in the form of DNA or RNA, into a cell in order to alter the pattern of gene expression in that cell.

genetic variant. A variation in an individual's genes, such as an alteration in DNA sequence, that may or may not have an apparent effect on the person's health, observable characteristics, or traits.

genome. All of an organism's hereditary information encoded in DNA and RNA.

genomics. The study of all of the genes in a cell or an organism.

glucose. A type of sugar present in the blood. It is the primary source of energy for the body's cells.

heart block. A condition in which conduction of the heart's electrical impulses is blocked or slowed along its normal pathway.

heart failure. A condition in which the heart's pumping is inadequate to meet the body's needs.

heart-lung machine. See **cardiopulmonary bypass.**

heart murmur. An extra or unusual sound heard during the heartbeat.

heparin. An anticoagulant drug that is administered intravenously or by injection.

high-density lipoprotein cholesterol (HDL-C). The cholesterol contained in **high-density lipoproteins,** which are lipoproteins in the blood that are believed to return excess cholesterol to the liver for excretion. HDL-C is known as the "good" cholesterol because high levels correlate with reduced risk for coronary artery disease.

Holter® monitor. May also be called **ambulatory electrocardiography.** A portable electrocardiography device that is worn outside of the doctor's office to detect possible arrhythmias.

homocysteine. An amino acid; elevated levels can predispose blood factors to form clots and are linked to increased risk for heart attack and stroke.

hypercholesterolemia. Elevation in total cholesterol and/or LDL-C levels.

hypertension. A condition in which the blood pressure within the arteries is elevated.

hypertriglyceridemia. Elevation in triglyceride levels.

hypotension. Abnormally low blood pressure.

imaging, medical. Refers to various techniques that allow visualization of the body's interior organs and tissues. May be used for diagnostic and therapeutic purposes.

implantable cardioverter-defibrillator (ICD). A battery-powered device implanted within the chest that is capable of both pacing the heart when abnormal rhythms occur and delivering a shock to it to convert abnormal rhythms (ventricular fibrillation and tachycardia) to normal ones.

infarction. An area of dead tissue resulting from obstruction of the artery supplying that area.

infective endocarditis. Inflammation of the endocardium (the inner membrane lining the heart) caused by bacteria. Both a potential cause and a complication of valvular disease.

inflammation. In reference to atherosclerosis, a state within the arterial wall that is especially conducive to plaque growth and rupture. C-reactive protein is a marker of inflammation in atherosclerosis.

insulin resistance. A state in which the hormone **insulin** becomes less effective at lowering glucose levels in the blood. It can lead to the development of type II diabetes.

intermediate-density lipoprotein (IDL). Lipoprotein formed from very low-density lipoprotein that may then be converted to low-density lipoprotein. Can contribute to the development of atherosclerosis.

intermittent claudication. Excessive fatigue or pain in the buttocks, thighs, or calves of the legs produced by exertion, such as walking, and relieved by a brief period of rest. A symptom of peripheral artery disease.

intima. The innermost layer of the artery wall that is in contact with the blood.

intravascular ultrasound (IVUS). An imaging technique using ultrasound during cardiac catheterization that provides a cross-sectional view of an artery, including atherosclerotic plaque growth within it.

ischemia. Deficiency in the normal supply of blood and oxygen to an area. Myocardial ischemia is deficiency in the flow of blood to the heart.

ischemic. The state in which a cell or tissue has an insufficient supply of blood, for instance in ischemic heart disease and ischemic stroke.

left ventricular dysfunction. A condition in which the pumping function of the left ventricle of the heart (responsible for pumping blood to the rest of the body) becomes impaired. Can lead to heart failure.

lipid profile. Includes measures of total cholesterol, HDL-C, triglyceride, and LDL-C. Triglyceride measurements are only accurate after fasting.

lipids. Fatty substances, including cholesterol, triglyceride, and phospholipid, that are present in the blood and tissues.

lipid triad. See atherogenic dyslipidemia.

lipoprotein(a). Also called Lp(a). A lipoprotein identical to LDL except for the addition of a special protein called apolipoprotein(a). Elevations of lipoprotein(a) are linked to increased cardiovascular risk.

lipoproteins. Macromolecules consisting of lipids and proteins that transport cholesterol (mostly as cholesteryl ester) in the blood.

low-density lipoprotein cholesterol (LDL-C). The cholesterol contained in low-density lipoproteins (LDL), which are lipoproteins that carry most of the cholesterol in the blood and that are primarily involved in the development of atherosclerosis. LDL-C is known as the "bad" cholesterol because elevated levels increase the risk for coronary artery disease.

lumen. The inner space of an artery.

macrophage. A specialized white blood cell capable of consuming other cells or parts of cells. In the developing atherosclerotic plaque, it ingests LDL and becomes a foam cell.

magnetic resonance imaging (MRI). A noninvasive diagnostic technique that uses radio waves within a magnetic field to produce computerized images of internal structures.

media. The middle, elastic layer of the arterial wall capable of constriction and relaxation and containing smooth muscle cells.

metabolic syndrome. A cluster of cardiovascular risk factors, including abdominal obesity, high blood pressure, elevated triglycerides, low HDL-C, elevated glucose levels, inflammation, and/or increased blood clotting. It increases risk for diabetes and coronary heart disease.

minimally invasive surgery. As opposed to open-heart surgery in which the breastbone is divided, it is a type of surgery involving smaller incisions in the chest. Includes **port-access surgery.**

mitral regurgitation. Dysfunction of the mitral valve, which allows blood to flow back into the left atrium.

mitral stenosis. Narrowing of the mitral valve.

mitral valve. Also called **bicuspid valve.** The valve separating the left atrium from the left ventricle of the heart.

mitral valve prolapse. A valvular abnormality characterized by a "floppy" mitral valve with leaflets that balloon backwards into the atrium like a parachute opening. May cause mitral regurgitation, but may be benign.

monocyte. A type of white blood cell that plays a role in the atherosclerotic process by entering into the arterial wall and becoming a macrophage.

myocardial infarction. Used synonymously with **heart attack.** Refers to the death of part of the heart muscle, most often due to atherosclerotic plaque blockage in the coronary arteries or a blood clot.

myocardial perfusion. The delivery of nutrients and oxygen in the blood to heart tissue.

myopathy. Muscular disease that is a potential side effect of statin therapy. Characterized by muscle pain, soreness, or weakness and elevations in creatine kinase.

nicotine replacement therapy. Various over-the-counter and prescription medications, including nicotine patches, gum, nasal sprays, inhalers, and lozenges, that help people to stop smoking by alleviating symptoms of nicotine withdrawal.

nicotinic acid. A drug used to raise HDL-C levels and decrease triglycerides; it also reduces LDL-C and Lp(a) levels. It works by decreasing the production of VLDL by the liver, which affects the levels of other lipoproteins. Not related to nicotine.

nitrates. A class of drugs, including nitroglycerin, that widen blood vessels and are used to treat angina.

non-HDL-C. A measure of "bad" cholesterol that can be calculated by subtracting the HDL-C level from the total cholesterol level.

non-ST-elevation myocardial infarction (NSTEMI). A type of heart attack in which electrocardiography tests indicate that the coronary arteries are most likely only partially blocked. Considered an acute coronary syndrome.

nuclear imaging. Various methods of producing three-dimensional images of the heart's blood flow, structure, and function by injecting radioactive tracers, called radionuclides, into the bloodstream. Includes single photon emission computed tomography and positron emission tomography.

oral glucose tolerance test (OGTT). A blood test for diagnosing diabetes that determines how quickly the body clears glucose from the system after the patient drinks a glucose solution. People with **impaired glucose tolerance** have prediabetes and are at increased risk for developing diabetes.

oxidation. As it relates to atherosclerosis, a chemical modification that occurs to LDL particles that makes them more damaging to the arterial wall and promotes atherosclerotic plaque development.

pacemaker, artificial. A mechanical device implanted in the chest that can be used to maintain a normal heart rate.

palpitation. A subjective feeling of an irregular or rapid heartbeat.

pancreatitis. The potentially life-threatening inflammation of the pancreas. Triglyceride levels above 1000 mg/dL increase risk for pancreatitis.

paroxysmal nocturnal dyspnea. A nighttime attack of breathing difficulty.

percutaneous coronary intervention (PCI). Also known as **percutaneous transluminal coronary angioplasty (PTCA).** A procedure to unblock clogged coronary arteries using a catheter. It may include **balloon angioplasty** (inflation of a small balloon to crack atherosclerotic plaque and stretch open the vessel wall), **atherectomy** (removal of plaque), and **stent placement.**

percutaneous intervention. A medical procedure that provides access to organs or tissues through a needle puncture in the skin, as opposed to a surgical procedure that requires the opening of the body with a scalpel.

peripheral artery disease. An atherosclerotic disease that develops in the arms or legs.

personalized medicine. A model for medical care that would incorporate information about a person's genetic makeup into all stages of prevention, diagnosis, and treatment.

phospholipid. A complex lipid that is a component of both cell membranes and lipoproteins.

plasma. The fluid component of the blood.

platelet aggregation. Activation and clumping of platelets (small cells carried in the blood) prior to clot formation.

pluripotent stem cells. Stem cells capable of differentiating, under the right conditions, into any other kind of cell normally found in an adult organism. **Induced pluripotent cells** are adult body cells that have been reprogrammed to resemble pluripotent stem cells.

positron emission tomography (PET). An imaging technique that provides a three-dimensional image by measuring the gamma radiation emitted when electrons in cells collide with positrons from radioactive tracers. Used to evaluate myocardial perfusion (blood flow to the heart) and to distinguish between dead areas of heart tissue and tissue capable of functioning again.

prediabetes. A state in which blood glucose levels are elevated but not high enough for a diagnosis of diabetes. Defined as having impaired glucose tolerance or impaired fasting glucose.

primary prevention. Strategies to prevent a first occurrence of a disease both in specific individuals and in the population at large.

proteoglycans. Molecules that provide structural support within the arterial wall. It is hypothesized that the first step in the atherosclerotic process occurs when apolipoprotein B particles in LDL bind to proteoglycans, causing LDL to become trapped in the arterial wall.

proteomics. The study of all of the proteins in a cell or in an organism.

pulmonary edema. A condition associated with heart failure in which fluid accumulates in and around the lungs.

pulmonary valve. The valve between the right ventricle and the pulmonary artery.

regression. In reference to atherosclerosis, an improvement in the disease as indicated by an increase in the diameter of a narrowed artery or a decrease in plaque size. Clinical trials have shown slowed progression and regression of atherosclerotic disease with lipid lowering.

regurgitation. As it refers to valvular disease, failure of the valves to fully close such that blood flows backward between heart chambers. Also called **insufficiency** or **incompetence.**

renin. An enzyme in the kidney that helps regulate fluid balance and blood vessel contraction.

restenosis. Reclosing of a blood vessel after it has been unblocked by percutaneous intervention.

revascularization. Restoration of blood flow through an artery blocked by a clot or by atherosclerotic plaque.

reverse cholesterol transport. The process in which HDL draws cholesterol out of macrophages in a growing atherosclerotic plaque and transports it back to the liver for disposal. Believed to be a major property of HDL, the "good" cholesterol.

rhabdomyolysis. A form of muscle disease in which muscle fibers break down. A very rare potential side effect of statin therapy.

risk factor. A trait or habit that helps predict the probability that a person will develop a particular disease; may be genetic or related to lifestyle or environment.

saturated fat. A fat found in foods of animal origin, as well as in palm, coconut, and palm kernel oils. It is the primary dietary factor that raises total cholesterol and LDL-C levels.

secondary prevention. Strategies to prevent the recurrence of a disease.

sick sinus syndrome. A set of heart rhythm abnormalities related to the failure of the sinoatrial node to perform its pacemaker duties satisfactorily.

single-nucleotide polymorphism (SNP). A type of genetic variant in which there is a substitution of just one base (a component of a nucleotide) in a DNA sequence.

single photo emission computed tomography (SPECT). An imaging technique that provides a three-dimensional image by measuring the gamma radiation emitted from radioactive tracers. May be used to evaluate myocardial perfusion.

sinoatrial (SA) node. Also called the **sinus node.** The body's natural pacemaker; a small bundle of muscle fibers and nerves within the wall of the right atrium that sends out electrical impulses at regular intervals and causes the heart to contract.

small dense LDL. Type of LDL particle associated with increased risk for heart disease. Often found in patients with low HDL-C and high triglycerides (atherogenic dyslipidemia).

statins. Short name for **HMG-CoA reductase inhibitors**, a class of drugs used primarily to lower LDL-C (currently includes atorvastatin, fluvastatin, lovastatin, pitavastatin, pravastatin, rosuvastatin, and simvastatin). Also have beneficial effects on other lipids and have been shown to reduce the risk of future cardiovascular events.

ST-elevation myocardial infarction (STEMI). A type of heart attack in which electrocardiography tests indicate that a coronary artery is most likely completely blocked. Requires immediate revascularization.

stem cell therapy. Future application of current stem cell research to treat human diseases. Could take the form of introducing stem cells to areas damaged by disease and stimulating the growth of new body cells.

stenosis. As it refers to atherosclerosis, the narrowing of an artery due to plaque growth. As it refers to valvular disease, the narrowing of the opening through a valve.

stent. A thin mesh tube made out of metal that may be inserted in an artery during percutaneous intervention and left within the blood vessel permanently to prevent it from reclosing.

steroid. A group of chemical compounds that includes cholesterol and the reproductive hormones progesterone, estrogen, and testosterone.

stroke. Also called **cerebrovascular disease.** An interruption in blood flow to the brain due to a clot (ischemic stroke) or hemorrhage.

subclinical atherosclerosis. Atherosclerotic disease that has been detected by tests but that does not cause symptoms such as chest pain (asymptomatic) and has not yet led to a coronary event.

sudden cardiac death. Unexpected death from cardiac causes, typically occurring within one hour of the start of symptoms. It can result from any heart condition and is not the same as cardiac arrest or a heart attack, although both of these conditions can lead to sudden cardiac death. Most sudden cardiac deaths are caused by arrhythmias, in particular ventricular fibrillation.

supraventricular tachycardia. Also called **atrial tachycardia**. A sustained rapid heartbeat that originates in the atria or the atrioventricular node.

syncope. Fainting or loss of consciousness.

systole. The phase of the heart's cycle during which the heart muscle contracts to pump blood to the body.

systolic blood pressure. The higher number in a blood pressure reading, observed during systole when the ventricles contract.

systolic heart failure. A type of heart failure caused by inability of the heart to contract fully and expel blood into the circulation.

tachycardia. A fast resting heart rate, more than one hundred beats per minute.

thrombin. A protein involved in blood clotting. It stimulates platelet aggregation and generates fibrin, which binds the platelets together.

thrombolytic therapy. Also called **fibrinolytic therapy**. Drugs that dissolve blood clots that may have blocked blood flow to the heart during a heart attack, to the brain during an ischemic stroke, or to the limbs during critical limb ischemia.

thrombosis. The formation of a blood clot. When it occurs in the arteries, it can cause a heart attack or stroke.

thrombus. A clot in a blood vessel or in one of the cavities of the heart.

total cholesterol. A measure of all of the cholesterol and triglycerides in the blood, including LDL-C, HDL-C, and other lipids.

transient ischemic attack (TIA). A ministroke, characterized by stroke symptoms generally lasting less than five minutes and causing no permanent damage.

translational research. A model for biomedical research that aims to speed the transition between laboratory findings and clinical applications (patient care).

tricuspid valve. The valve between the right atrium and the right ventricle, so called because it has three cusps.

triglyceride. A primary component of animal fats and vegetable oils. Triglycerides store energy in the body as fat.

type A personality. A competitive, aggressive, and time-pressured personality type. Studies have not demonstrated that it is associated with increased risk of heart disease.

type D personality. Personality type characterized by negative emotions such as worry, anxiety, and pessimism and by emotional and social inhibition. Research into its relationship to heart disease is ongoing.

type I diabetes. Also called **insulin-dependent diabetes mellitus.** A form of diabetes that usually develops suddenly in childhood or adolescence and is characterized by a total lack of insulin in the body.

type II diabetes. Also called **non-insulin-dependent diabetes mellitus.** A form of diabetes that develops gradually and is characterized by insulin resistance. Associated with obesity.

ultrafast computed tomography (CT). A very fast scanning method often used to detect calcium deposits in the coronary arteries.

vagal nerve stimulation. Attempts to slow the heart rate during episodes of arrhythmia by stimulating the vagus nerves, which extend from the brain to the abdomen and help regulate the function of various organs.

valves. Tissues in the passageways between the atria and ventricles that control the passage of blood.

valvular disease. A dysfunction or abnormality of the heart valves.

valvuloplasty. Also called **valvotomy.** A procedure to widen a blocked valve opening. May be percutaneous or surgical.

vasa vasorum. A network of small blood vessels that supply oxygen to the outer wall of larger arteries and veins.

vascular. Pertaining to the blood vessels of the body.

vasoconstriction. The muscular contraction of the walls of an artery. Can be due to the effects of atherosclerosis.

vasodilator. A drug or substance that relaxes and widens blood vessels.

ventricles. The lower chambers of the heart from which blood is propelled out to the lungs and the rest of the body.

ventricular assist devices (VAD). Some may also be called **left ventricular assist devices (LVAD).** Machines that support the function of the heart by helping it to pump blood. Consist of external devices used in the hospital and smaller, portable devices that can be partially or totally implanted in the body.

ventricular fibrillation. A heart irregularity or arrhythmia in which the ventricles beat very fast but ineffectively such that blood is not pumped out to supply the body. This condition results in cardiac arrest and death if not treated immediately.

ventricular tachycardia. A sustained, rapid, and regular heartbeat that arises in the ventricles. Can potentially lead to ventricular fibrillation.

very low-density lipoprotein (VLDL). A lipoprotein produced by the liver that delivers triglyceride to cells. A fasting lipid profile measures the total amount of triglyceride contained in VLDL particles.

vulnerable plaque. A type of atherosclerotic lesion that is highly prone to rupture and is the most common cause of coronary events. It has a lipid-rich core encased by a thin fibrous cap, and it may narrow arteries by 30 to 50 percent.

INDEX

Pages in **bold** indicate figures and illustrations.

291